Medicine

NOTICE

Medicine is an ever-changing science. As new research and clinical experience broaden our knowledge, changes in treatment and drug therapy are required. The editors and the publisher of this work have checked with sources believed to be reliable in their efforts to provide information that is complete and generally in accord with the standards accepted at the time of publication. However, in view of the possibility of human error or changes in medical sciences, neither the editors, nor the publisher, nor any other party who has been involved in the preparation or publication of this work warrants that the information contained herein is in every respect accurate or complete. Readers are encouraged to confirm the information contained herein with other sources. For example and in particular, readers are advised to check the product information sheet included in the package of each drug they plan to administer to be certain that the information contained in this book is accurate and that changes have not been made in the recommended dose or in the contraindications for administration. This recommendation is of particular importance in connection with new or infrequently used drugs.

Medicine
PreTest® Self-Assessment and Review

Fifth Edition

Edited by

Amos Bodner, M.D.
Vice President
Pediatric Pharmaceuticals
Edison, New Jersey

McGraw-Hill Information Services Company
Health Professions Division
PreTest Series

New York   St. Louis   San Francisco   Colorado Springs   Auckland   Bogotá   Hamburg
Lisbon   London   Madrid   Mexico   Milan   Montreal   New Delhi   Panama   Paris
San Juan   São Paulo   Singapore   Sydney   Tokyo   Toronto

Library of Congress Cataloging-in-Publication Data

Medicine : PreTest self-assessment and review. — 5th ed. / edited by
   Amos Bodner.
         p.   cm. — (Clinical sciences series)
   Bibliography: p.
   ISBN 0–07–051969–2 : $14.95 (est.)
   1. Medicine—Examinations, questions, etc.   2. National Board of
Medical Examiners—Examinations—Study guides.   3. Federation of
State Medical Boards of the United States—Examinations—Study
guides.   4. Educational Commission for Foreign Medical Graduates—
Examinations—Study guides.   I. Bodner, Amos.   II. Series.
   [DNLM: 1. Medicine—examination questions.   W 18 M4914]
R834.5.M4   1989
616'.0076—dc19
DNLM/DLC
for Library of Congress   88–37042
                                                                          CIP

This book was set in Times Roman by Waldman Graphics, Inc.; the editors
were J. Dereck Jeffers and Bruce MacGregor; the production supervisor was
Clara B. Stanley.
R.R. Donnelley & Sons was printer and binder.

   1 2 3 4 5 6 7 8 9 0   DOCDOC   8 9 4 3 2 1 0 9

ISBN 0–07–051969–2

Contents

Preface

A wide base of fundamental knowledge is essential to clinical competence. Because medicine is evolving in logarithmic fashion, self-assessment is, by necessity, a perpetual process. This book is primarily an educational tool and its goal is to aid physicians in targeting those areas of medicine that require more attention.

For this edition, a substantial number of new questions have been provided and dated material has been replaced to parallel changes in clinical practice. The bibliography reflects an attempt to use the latest editions of standard textbooks and journals of progressive sophistication and is provided to allow for further study in those areas requiring review.

It is hoped that as we acquire information our ability to use that knowledge in a compassionate, professional, and ethical manner will grow as well. For while aspects of medicine may change, the principle of beneficence, of assisting others in need and avoiding harm, never will.

A.B.

Introduction

Medicine, PreTest Self-Assessment and Review, 5th Ed., has been designed to provide medical students, as well as physicians, with a comprehensive and convenient instrument for self-assessment and review within the field of medicine. The 500 questions provided have been designed to parallel the format and degree of difficulty of the questions contained in Part II of the National Board of Medical Examiners examinations, the Federation Licensing Examination (FLEX), and the Foreign Medical Graduate Examination in the Medical Sciences (FMGEMS).

Each question in the book is accompanied by an answer, a paragraph explanation, and a specific page reference to either a current journal article, a textbook, or both. A bibliography that lists all the sources used in the book follows the last chapter.

Perhaps the most effective way to use this book is to allow yourself one minute to answer each question in a given chapter; as you proceed, indicate your answer beside each question. By following this suggestion, you will be approximating the time limits imposed by the board examinations previously mentioned.

When you have finished answering the questions in a chapter, you should then spend as much time as you need verifying your answers and carefully reading the explanations. Although you should pay special attention to the explanations for the questions you answered incorrectly, you should read every explanation. The authors of this book have designed the explanations to reinforce and supplement the information tested by the questions. If, after reading the explanations for a given chapter, you feel you need still more information about the material covered, you should consult and study the references indicated.

Medicine

Allergy and Immunology

DIRECTIONS: Each question below contains five suggested responses. Select the **one best** response to each question.

1. Which of the following statements about the administration and use of intravenous gammaglobulin is correct?

(A) The administration of high doses may produce a remission in idiopathic thrombocytopenic purpura
(B) It must be administered slowly, as concentrated gammaglobulin used intravenously has spontaneous anticomplementary activity
(C) Intravenous gammaglobulin preparations are safe and effective in the management of patients with selective IgA deficiency
(D) Intravenous gammaglobulin preparations have been associated with the development of acquired immune deficiency syndrome (AIDS)
(E) In calculating the dose of intravenous gammaglobulin to be administered, the physician should take into account the fact that the half-life of the immunoglobulin in the product is 7 to 12 days in vivo

2. The majority of influenza epidemics in the U.S. have resulted in 10,000 to 20,000 excess deaths, primarily in persons with chronic pulmonary, renal, cardiovascular, metabolic, or immunologic diseases. Because of this, influenza vaccine is recommended for these high-risk people. Each of the following statements concerning influenza vaccines is true EXCEPT

(A) whole-virus vaccines are more immunogenic than split-product vaccines
(B) the vaccine should be administered during the fall of the year
(C) nonswine influenza vaccines have been associated with an increased risk of the Landry-Guillain-Barré syndrome
(D) a person not having received an annual influenza vaccine should be placed on amantadine hydrochloride
(E) children under 12 should receive the split-product vaccine owing to the high frequency of febrile reactions associated with the whole-virus vaccines

3. The presence of bacteria in endocardial vegetations in cases of infective endocarditis stimulates the immune system to produce nonspecific antibodies. True statements concerning this phenomenon include all the following EXCEPT

(A) higher concentrations of circulatory immune complexes correlate with extracardiac manifestations
(B) 50 percent of patients develop rheumatoid factor
(C) lowest levels of hemolytic complement are found in cases with associated immune complex glomerulonephritis
(D) antisarcolemmal antibodies are rarely found in patients with subacute bacterial endocarditis
(E) false positive tests for syphilis occasionally occur

4. Immunoglobulins prepared from pooled human plasma are available for prophylaxis against the development of hepatitis A and hepatitis B. True statements concerning the use of immunoglobulins in viral hepatitis include all the following EXCEPT

(A) immune globulin should be administered to staffs of daycare centers that care for diapered children and in which hepatitis A transmission has been documented
(B) routine immune globulin prophylaxis against hepatitis A is not indicated for hospital personnel
(C) travelers from the U.S. to high-risk areas outside ordinary tourist routes should receive immune globulin prophylaxis against hepatitis A
(D) needle-stick exposure to blood known to contain HBsAg requires a single dose of 0.02 ml/kg body weight hepatitis B immune globulin given immediately
(E) hepatitis B immune globulin given at birth to infants born to HBsAg-positive mothers prevents the carrier state in 75 percent of cases

5. Selective IgA deficiency is the most common of all immunodeficiency states. Study of patients who have this problem has revealed that

(A) they may suffer anaphylactic reactions following the administration of serum products
(B) clinical improvement follows regular infusions of fresh plasma
(C) secretory component is usually increased in an attempt to compensate for lack of secretory IgA
(D) there is an increase in 19S IgM in the secretions of certain affected patients
(E) a few of them have associated autoimmune disorders

6. Which of the following statements about assessment of immunoglobulin in cerebrospinal fluid is true?

(A) It may aid in the diagnosis of cerebral systemic lupus erythematosus
(B) It may lead to a suspicion of multiple sclerosis if IgM levels are elevated
(C) It may distinguish subacute sclerosing panencephalitis from multiple sclerosis
(D) It normally reveals that 5 to 10 percent of the cerebrospinal fluid protein is IgG
(E) It becomes more useful if the total cerebrospinal fluid protein exceeds 100 mg/100 ml

7. During the primary immune response a network of interactions is required for the successful elimination of antigen. During this process, which of the following occurs?

(A) T8 positive lymphocytes stimulate macrophages to release interleukin 2
(B) T4 positive lymphocytes stimulate macrophages to release interleukin 1
(C) B lymphocytes react with antigen and interleukin 1 and then secrete immunoglobulin M
(D) Antigen-presenting macrophages present antigens to lymphocyte-activating macrophages
(E) IgA antibodies are secreted by plasma cells that have interacted with secretory piece

8. In regard to the presence of circulating antideoxyribonucleoprotein in the serum of patients who have systemic lupus erythematosus, which of the following statements is true?

(A) It is associated with the presence of LE cells
(B) It is associated with leukopenia
(C) It is rarely associated with high titers of antinuclear factor
(D) Severe membranous glomerulonephritis is likely to be present
(E) It is unusual inasmuch as this antibody generally is associated with scleroderma

9. Which of the following statements about allergic reactions in patients receiving up to 20 g of penicillin per day is true?

(A) Allergic reactions occur in 20 percent of patients receiving the drug for the second time

(B) Allergic reactions may be anaphylactoid if IgE class antibodies to penicilloyl-P are present in the serum

(C) Allergic reactions will be less likely to occur if IgM antipenicilloyl antibodies are present in the serum

(D) Allergic reactions are unlikely to be anaphylactoid if the patient does not get a wheal and flare reaction when penicilloyl-D-lysine is introduced intradermally

(E) Allergic reactions can be complicated by hemolytic anemias when prolonged administration provokes the development of red blood cell autoantibodies

10. A 55-year-old farmer develops recurrent cough, dyspnea, fever, and myalgia several hours after entering his barn. All the following statements concerning this patient are true EXCEPT

(A) pulmonary function testing several hours after an exposure will most likely reveal a restrictive pattern

(B) immediate type IgE hypersensitivity is not involved in the pathogenesis of his illness

(C) the etiologic agents may well be thermophilic actinomycete antigens

(D) demonstrating precipitable antibodies to the offending antigen confirms the diagnosis of hypersensitivity pneumonitis

(E) a suppressor-cell functional defect is present

11. A 40-year-old man presents with a 3 month history of headache, sinusitis, and rhinorrhea. He has had two episodes of hemoptysis and some respiratory discomfort. On examination, he has some nasal mucosal ulcerations. His blood urea nitrogen is 60 mg per 100 ml. A biopsy of the swollen tissue in the patient's nose yields results consistent with the diagnosis of Wegener's granulomatosis. All the following histological features can be expected to be associated with this condition EXCEPT

(A) vasculitis affecting the small arterioles

(B) vasculitis involving venules and some capillaries

(C) deposition in blood vessels of immunoglobulin and, possibly, immune complexes

(D) necrotizing inflammation in which all affected vessels show the same degree of inflammation

(E) numerous giant cells in granulomata

12. All the following statements concerning the immunologic features of active sarcoidosis are true EXCEPT

(A) there are increased levels of circulating suppressor T lymphocytes

(B) patients exhibit cutaneous anergy

(C) the hypergammaglobulinemia is associated with circulating free light chains

(D) lymphocytosis is characteristic

(E) there are increased numbers of circulating B lymphocytes

13. An immunologic basis for atopic dermatitis is suggested by the fact that the majority of patients have a family history of other atopic disorders. Which of the following statements concerning this disease is true?

(A) It is ruled out by normal serum IgE levels

(B) Patients are susceptible to infection with herpes simplex and vaccinia

(C) Cell-mediated immune function is normal

(D) Total CH_{50} correlates with disease activity

(E) There is a higher incidence of contact dermatitis from poison ivy

14. A 15-year-old girl presents with a clinical syndrome that is indistinguishable from viral hepatitis; however, her history and serological findings do not support a viral etiology for her problem. Liver biopsy reveals an established active cirrhosis and hepatocellular necrosis associated with a heavy infiltrate of plasma cells and lymphocytes. Which of the following statements about this girl's condition is most likely to be true?

(A) B lymphocytes are likely to carry the histocompatibility antigen B7

(B) She probably has a total immunoglobulin level that exceeds 4 g/100 ml

(C) She probably has antimitochondrial antibodies

(D) High titers of anti–smooth muscle antibodies are likely to appear transiently at the onset of her illness

(E) She will probably recover spontaneously after 6 months of illness

15. A 6-year-old white male presents to his physician with a history of recurrent staphylococcal infections (including osteomyelitis), chronic severe eczema, and asthma complicated by allergic rhinitis. If the boy has the hyper-IgE syndrome, it is likely that

(A) his IgE level (normally less than 300 ng/ml) will be between 2000 and 5000 ng/ml
(B) his father will have suffered from similar problems as a child
(C) a chemotactic defect of polymorphonuclear cells will be discovered
(D) he will respond well to levamisole
(E) a B-cell, but not a T-cell, defect will be demonstrable

DIRECTIONS: Each question below contains four suggested responses of which **one or more** is correct. Select

A	if	**1, 2, and 3**	are correct
B	if	**1 and 3**	are correct
C	if	**2 and 4**	are correct
D	if	**4**	is correct
E	if	**1, 2, 3, and 4**	are correct

16. Correct statements about cryoglobulins include which of the following?

(1) They cannot activate the complement cascade
(2) They are found in most normal people
(3) They are rarely demonstrable in patients with biliary cirrhosis
(4) Clinical symptoms include palpable purpura and peripheral ulcers

17. A 15-year-old boy develops painless hematuria, myalgias, and malaise immediately following a viral upper respiratory infection. Renal biopsy reveals a focal and segmental proliferative glomerulonephritis with mesangial matrix increase and hypercellularity; immunofluorescence reveals diffuse staining for IgA and C3 in all mesangial areas. True statements about this boy's condition include that

(1) depressed levels of C3 and C4 are commonly found
(2) subendothelial and subepithelial deposits are associated with more severe disease
(3) early steroid therapy alters the natural history of the illness
(4) after 25 years, 50 percent of patients will have developed end-stage renal disease

18. Antibodies that act as circulating anticoagulants demonstrate which of the following characteristics?

(1) They usually are IgM in character
(2) They increase rapidly in the serum after exposure to blood or blood products
(3) They may be present for years in apparently normal postpartum women
(4) In patients who have systemic lupus erythematosus, they are often directed against activated factor X

19. True statements regarding immunological and inflammatory responses to glucocorticoid therapy include which of the following?

(1) There are fewer infectious complications with alternate-day therapy than with daily steroid therapy
(2) Reactivation of tuberculosis occurs with increased frequency in patients on chronic steroid therapy
(3) High-dose steroid therapy causes a decrease in immunoglobulin levels
(4) Permanent damage to the immunological system occurs with long-term steroid therapy

20. Allergic bronchopulmonary aspergillosis is associated with which of the following statements?

(1) Twenty-five percent of sputum cultures are negative for *Aspergillus fumigatus*
(2) It may lead to pulmonary fibrosis if left untreated
(3) Sputum and blood eosinophilia are characteristic
(4) IgE levels fluctuate with disease activity

21. Bone marrow–derived B lymphocytes exhibit which of the following characteristics?

(1) They are the proliferating cells in chronic lymphocytic leukemia
(2) They carry a surface membrane receptor for the Fc portion of IgG
(3) They carry a surface membrane receptor for the breakdown products of the third component of complement
(4) They have a receptor for the Epstein-Barr virus

22. Correct statements about multiple sclerosis (MS) include which of the following?

(1) Suppression of CSF immunoglobulin production leaves the central nervous system vulnerable to viral infection
(2) Suppressor T cells are drastically reduced in the blood of patients experiencing an acute flare-up of MS
(3) Oligoclonal binding in CSF is virtually diagnostic for MS, as it otherwise occurs only in the easily distinguished cryptococcal meningitis
(4) More than 50 percent of MS patients can be shown to be synthesizing antibody to the measles virus in their brain

23. Rheumatoid factors are autoantibodies that are associated with a wide variety of disease states. True statements concerning rheumatoid factors include that

(1) they are usually IgM directed against the Fc portion of IgG
(2) positivity in high titer correlates with an increased incidence of vasculitis in rheumatoid arthritis
(3) positivity increases with age
(4) salmonellosis is associated with a positive rheumatoid factor test

24. A 24-year-old woman has a severe anaphylactic reaction following a honeybee sting. She recovers, but is surprised and disappointed at her reaction since she had completed a course of desensitization with whole-body extract. In discussing the future management of this problem, the physician would be correct in telling the patient that

(1) she should have a skin test with whole-body extract and, if the result is positive, she should try a second course of desensitizing injections with this antigenic preparation

(2) she should not be alarmed about the situation because, despite the fact that there are hundreds of thousands of bee stings a year in the United States, only 50 to 60 deaths are reported annually

(3) even if she is stung after another course of desensitization and no immediate reaction occurs, she should watch for a delayed reaction for 6 hours after the sting

(4) most reactions appear to occur because of sensitivity to bee and hornet venom

DIRECTIONS: Each group of questions below consists of lettered headings followed by a set of numbered items. For each numbered item select the **one** lettered heading with which it is **most** closely associated. Each lettered heading may be used **once, more than once, or not at all.**

Questions 25–27

For each of the following immunological diseases select the component of the immune response that is most likely to be abnormal in that disease.

    (A) C1q
    (B) Inducer T cells
    (C) C3
    (D) Antigen-presenting macrophages
    (E) Gamma interferon

25. Acquired immune deficiency syndrome (AIDS)

26. Sex-linked agammaglobulinemia

27. Transient hypogammaglobulinemia of infancy

Questions 28–31

For each of the following disorders, select the feature with which it is mostly closely associated.

    (A) C1 esterase inhibitor
    (B) Peyer's patches
    (C) Rheumatoid factor
    (D) Allergic reactions to iodides
    (E) Sympathetic ophthalmia

28. Rheumatoid arthritis

29. Systemic lupus erythematosus

30. Sjögren's syndrome

31. Leprosy

DIRECTIONS: Each group of questions below consists of four lettered headings followed by a set of numbered items. For each numbered item select

A	if the item is associated with	(A) **only**
B	if the item is associated with	(B) **only**
C	if the item is associated with	**both** (A) and (B)
D	if the item is associated with	**neither** (A) nor (B)

Each lettered heading may be used **once, more than once, or not at all.**

Questions 32–36

(A) Bullous pemphigoid
(B) Pemphigus vulgaris
(C) Both
(D) Neither

32. Acantholysis

33. Anti–basement membrane zone antibodies

34. Positive Nikolsky's sign

35. Treatment with immunosuppressive drugs

36. Autoimmune disorders

Questions 37–41

(A) Cyclophosphamide
(B) Cyclosporine
(C) Both
(D) Neither

37. Inhibition of interleukin-2 production

38. Sparing of macrophage activity

39. No demonstrable effect on B cells

40. Myelotoxicity

41. Inhibition of the elaboration of α-interferon

Allergy and Immunology

Answers

1. The answer is A. *(Braunwald, ed 11. p 1392. Pirossky, Am J Med Proc Symposium 3:53–56, 1984.)* The availability of concentrated forms of gammaglobulin suitable for intravenous use represents a significant advance in the management of immunodeficiency states. Immune serum globulin (ISG) could not be given intravenously, as the aggregates in the material have spontaneous anticomplementary activity and would cause an anaphylactic-like reaction; intravenous preparations of gammaglobulin do not have spontaneous anticomplementary activity but do retain the ability to activate the classical complement cascade after combining with antigen. Intravenous gammaglobulin can be administered to premature babies who have low immunoglobulin levels because of poor transplacental passage of maternal IgG. Apart from its obvious use in the management of congenital and acquired hypogammaglobulinemia, intravenous gammaglobulin provides the preferable way of replacing gammaglobulin for patients who are severely burned, who have hypergammaglobulinemia secondary to chronic lymphatic leukemia or multiple myeloma, and who need IgG after plasmapheresis. The product only contains trace amounts of IgA and is therefore not suitable for administration to patients who have a selective IgA deficiency. Such patients may well make IgE anti-IgA antibodies that could produce an immediate hypersensitivity reaction. The product is prepared from pooled plasma obtained at numerous collection sites, thus ensuring that antibodies to ubiquitous antigens are represented in each batch of the product. Neither AIDS nor hepatitis has been associated with its use. The half-life of the IgG in the product is approximately 27 days, so it can be administered on a monthly basis. Although the mechanisms are as yet unknown, it is of interest that high doses of intravenous gammaglobulin (1 g/kg over 5 days) will produce remission in both acute and chronic idiopathic thrombocytopenic purpura in many patients. In addition, its administration has led to remission in autoimmune neutropenia.

2. The answer is C. *(Braunwald, ed 11. p 528.)* Vaccination of high-risk populations has been shown to confer a 60 to 95 percent protection from the consequences of influenza. Influenza vaccines usually contain influenza A and influenza B prototype antigens of the prevalent circulating types of influenza virus. Either whole-virus or split-product vaccine may be used in adults; the former is more immunogenic but has a higher frequency of febrile reactions. The vaccines are administered during the fall of the year. While severe adverse reactions are uncommon, an excess risk of Landry-Guillain-Barré syndrome occurred in recipients of

A/New Jersey/76 swine influenza vaccine; approximately 10 cases for every one million vaccinated were recorded. This association does not exist for the more recent nonswine influenza vaccines. Patients in high-risk populations who have not received their annual influenza vaccine should be placed on 100 mg amantadine hydrochloride twice daily while influenza A is still identified regionally or until protection is conferred with receipt of the influenza vaccine.

3.   The answer is D. *(Hurst, ed 6. pp 1139–1140.)* While the symptoms of subacute endocarditis develop insidiously, the clinical and laboratory manifestations may be grouped under three categories: as evidence of a systemic infection, an intravascular lesion, or an immunologic reaction to infection. As noted, the presence of bacteria in endocardial vegetations stimulates the production of nonspecific antibodies leading to polyclonal increases in gamma globulins, positive rheumatoid factor, occasional false positive tests for syphilis, and decreased complement. Circulating immune complexes have been detected in the vast majority of patients; higher concentrations correlate with the presence of arthritis, splenomegaly, and glomerulonephritis. Antiendocardial and antisarcolemmal antibodies are found in 60 to 100 percent of cases. By history, manifestations of immunologic reactions include arthralgia, myalgia, and tenosynovitis; physical examination reveals arthritis, signs of uremia, vascular phenomena, and finger clubbing.

4.   The answer is D. *(Centers for Disease Control, Ann Intern Med 96:193–197, 1982.)* Immune globulins are sterile solutions of antibodies obtained from professional donors and contain antibodies against the hepatitis A virus and the hepatitis B surface antigen at stable titers. Hepatitis B immune globulin is prepared from plasma containing extremely high titers of anti-HBs. Hepatitis A is a common infection in the U.S.; more than half the population over 40 have serologic evidence of past infection. It has been confirmed that immune globulin given before exposure or during the incubation period of hepatitis A is protective, although the prophylactic value is greatest when given early in the incubation period. Postexposure prophylaxis for hepatitis A is recommended for all those in household and sexual contact with persons with hepatitis A; for the staffs of daycare centers in which HAV transmission is occurring; and for staffs of institutions for custodial care that have outbreaks of hepatitis A. The recommended dosage is 0.02 ml/kg body weight of immune globulin given as a single intramuscular dose. Preexposure prophylaxis is recommended for travelers to high-risk areas outside tourist routes. A single intramuscular dose of 0.02 ml/kg body weight is recommended unless travel is prolonged, in which case 0.06 ml/kg should be given every 5 months. For hepatitis B, recommendations are based on the following facts: hepatitis B immune globulin is preferable to immune globulin when percutaneous or mucous membrane exposure to blood known to contain HBsAg occurs; in the hospital the risk of clinical hepatitis B after exposure to blood known to contain HBsAg is 1 in 20; and if the blood is of unknown HBsAg status, the risk is 1 in 2000. Therefore, exposure to an HBsAg-positive source requires prophylaxis with hepatitis B immune globulin, 0.06 ml/kg body weight immediately and again 1 month later. Exposure to a source of unknown status but of a high-risk group requires HBsAg testing if results can be known within 7 days, and immune globulin .06 ml/kg body weight immediately; if the test is positive, hepatitis B immune globulin is given at that time and 1 month later, and if the test is negative, nothing need be done. For an exposure to a source of unknown status and of a low-risk group or unknown source, prophylaxis with .06 ml/kg body weight of immune globulin is optional. Preexposure prophylaxis with immune globulin .05 to .07 ml/kg body weight is recommended to staff and patients of hemodialysis units and institutions for custodial care if hygenic measures fail to stop transmission of hepatitis B.

5.   The answer is A. *(Braunwald, ed 11. p 1390.)* IgA deficiency occurs in approximately 1 out of 700 births. Failure to produce this antibody results in recurrent upper respiratory tract infections in 50 percent of affected patients. IgA-deficient patients frequently have autoimmune disorders, atopic problems, and malabsorption and eventually develop pulmonary disease. There is an increased incidence of malignancy in these cases. Replacement therapy is entirely unsatisfactory. If IgA is totally absent, its administration can represent an antigenic challenge that may result in anaphylaxis. Secretory component is normally present, and very few cases of IgA deficiency are due to a lack of this accessory factor. Some patients compensate for IgA deficiency by secreting a low-molecular-weight 7S IgM antibody.

6.   The answer is D. *(Braunwald, ed 11. pp 1997–1998.)* Normally, IgG represents 5 to 10 percent of the total protein in cerebrospinal fluid. Levels exceeding 12 percent have been shown to correlate with the presence of either multiple sclerosis or subacute sclerosing panencephalitis. In other conditions, evaluations of cerebrospinal fluid immunoglobulin have not been valuable because the IgG fraction usually remains proportionate to the total level of cerebrospinal fluid protein. The discriminatory value of IgG determination is lessened once the level of total protein exceeds 100 mg/100 ml.

7.   The answer is B. *(Braunwald, ed 11. pp 328–337. Paul, pp 562–568.)* The primary immune response involves an initial presentation of antigen to a T4 inducer cell by an antigen-presenting macrophage. The latter cell is remarkable for the strong expression of D locus-derived antigen on its membrane. The cell is thus able to present both foreignness and self to a T4 inducer cell, an essential step in initiating the immune response. Lymphocytes carrying the surface antigen T4 (detected by monoclonal antibodies) then activate a second class of macrophages known as lymphocyte-activating macrophages. This cell releases interleukin 1, a messenger substance that binds to a receptor on the surface of the T4 cell generated after the binding of antigen. The T4 cell, which has bound foreignness, self, and interleukin 1, releases interleukin 2, a soluble messenger substance that gives a vital permissive signal to those lymphocytes involved in the actual production of an inflammatory response that will eliminate antigen. Interleukin 2 binds to B cells that have recognized antigen and allows them to mature into plasma cells that will secrete antibody. The initial antibody secreted will be IgM in class. Interleukin 2 also binds to T cells capable of producing delayed-type hypersensitivity after exposure to antigen and to cytotoxic T cells that can kill a target cell after direct membrane interaction with antigen. The fact that T4 cells are a prime target for the agent responsible for the acquired immune deficiency syndrome explains the profound immunodeficiency that develops in such patients who lack the capacity to induce a successful immune response. Trials of interleukin 2 are under way for the treatment of both immunodeficiency and cancer.

8.   The answer is A. *(Braunwald, ed 11. pp 1418–1419.)* Antideoxyribonucleoprotein (anti-DNP) antibody, one of the antinuclear factors found in the lupus erythematosus (LE) cluster of diseases, constitutes the LE factor that promotes phagocytosis of nuclear material by polymorphonuclear leukocytes to produce the LE cell. While the antibody is associated with lupus erythematosus, it is not as good a correlate of renal disease as is the presence of antideoxyribonucleic acid antibody. Antibodies to soluble nuclear extracts correlate better with scleroderma. Although individuals who have systemic lupus erythematosus can exhibit leukopenia and even an antibody to neutrophils, such phenomena are not particularly associated with anti-DNP antibody.

9.   The answer is B. *(Braunwald, ed 11. pp 491–493, 1410–1411. Eisen, ed 2. pp 516–519.)* Allergic reactions to penicillin consist of (1) immediate hypersensitivity reactions; (2) delayed-immediate type hypersensitivity reactions; (3) delayed in-time reactions; and (4) delayed reactions involving organ-specific tissue. The antigenic determinants of penicillin that provoke these reactions can be subdivided into minor and major determinants. The major determinants constitute the majority of the breakdown metabolites of penicillin and are represented by the penicilloyl derivatives. It is the minor determinants, however, that produce most of the severe, immediate allergic reactions. Penicillin hypersensitivity is usually mediated by IgE and IgM antibodies against these metabolic degradation products of penicillin. With both the major and the minor determinants, it is necessary for the penicillin to form a conjugate with a body protein, inasmuch as the breakdown products of penicillin are not, in themselves, immunogenic. Such complexes are known as hapten protein conjugates. IgE antibody—usually against minor determinants—can produce the severe immediate anaphylactoid reactions that often are life threatening. Sensitivity to these minor determinants can only be predicted from a patient's history and from immediate hypersensitivity reactions to intradermal injection of the drug to be used. Minor determinant mixtures for skin testing are not commercially available. In some patients, however, IgE antibodies to the major (penicilloyl) determinants are present, and immediate hypersensitivity in the skin will occur following skin testing with penicilloyl. While most of the immediate (2 to 30 minutes) reactions are due to IgE antibody directed against minor determinants, reactions that begin within 3 hours and, perhaps, as late as 72 hours can be mediated by IgE against the penicilloyl derivatives. These are known as delayed-immediate hypersensitivity reactions. Delayed in-time reactions, which are mediated by IgG antibodies, occur after 48 hours. The majority of penicillin reactions are caused by complement activation following IgM antibodies combining with major determinants. The hapten protein complexes are usually formed in the skin, which, therefore, becomes a frequent target for the reaction, although serum sickness–like disease may occur. Hemolytic anemia can occur if penicillin determinants for hapten protein conjugate with red blood cells. Antipenicillin antibodies react with the adsorbed penicillin, causing subsequent red blood cell lysis. No autoantibodies are formed in this condition. Allergic reactions may occur in as many as 10 percent of persons treated with penicillin, and there seems little doubt that IgG blocking antibodies prevent an even higher incidence of such reactions.

10. The answer is D. *(Levy, Ann Allergy 54:167–171, 1985.)* Hypersensitivity pneumonitis is characterized by an immunologic inflammatory reaction in response to inhaling organic dusts, the most common of which are thermophilic actinomycetes, fungi, and avian proteins. In the acute form of the illness, exposure to the offending antigen is intense and cough, dyspnea, fever, chills, and myalgia, which typically occur 4 to 8 hours after exposure, are the presenting symptoms. In the subacute form, antigen exposure is moderate, chills and fever are usually absent, and cough, anorexia, weight loss, and dyspnea dominate the presentation. In the chronic form of hypersensitivity pneumonitis, progressive dyspnea, weight loss, and anorexia are seen; pulmonary fibrosis is a noted complication. In most cases, leukocytosis and eosinophilia are present; the finding of IgG antibody to the offending antigen is universal although it may be present in asymptomatic patients as well and is therefore not diagnostic. While peripheral T cell, B cell, and monocyte counts are normal, a suppressor-cell functional defect can be demonstrated in these patients. Inhalation challenge with the suspected antigen and concomitant pulmonary function testing help to confirm the diagnosis. Therapy involves avoidance; steroids are administered in severe cases. Bronchodilators and antihistamines are not effective.

11. The answer is D. *(Braunwald, ed 11. pp 1442–1443.)* Necrotizing vasculitis is associated with a variety of conditions that cover the spectrum from leukocytoclastic angiitis to necrotizing midline granuloma. Within this spectrum, a clinically definable constellation of clinical and pathological findings makes it possible to define the syndrome known as Wegener's granulomatosis. The therapeutic and prognostic implications of this syndrome make its diagnosis a matter of some importance. Wegener's granulomatosis is a systemic disease in which inflammation results from vasculitis occurring in many vessels throughout the body. Venules, capillaries, and arterioles are all affected in this disease, which is most commonly seen in men in the fourth and fifth decades of life. Characteristically, however, blood vessels in the kidneys and both upper and lower respiratory tracts are most affected. Although the evidence is not conclusive, there are data to suggest that the immune system produces this vasculitis as part of a hypersensitivity reaction to an antigenic encounter yet to be identified. Circulating immune complexes have been demonstrated in some, but not all, cases and granulomata are found in many tissues, observations that strengthen the concept of a hypersensitivity state and implicate cell-mediated immunity in the pathogenesis of the disease. Giant-cell formation, probably representing fused macrophages, is often associated with the granulomata. The vasculitis associated with Wegener's granulomatosis is unusual in that careful examination of blood vessels in one tissue section will show some that are undergoing early inflammatory changes, others that are obviously healing, and still others that are permanently sclerosed.

12. The answer is D. *(Rohatgi, Ann Allergy 52:316–325, 1984.)* Sarcoidosis is a multisystem granulomatous disorder characterized by bilateral hilar lymphadenopathy; pulmonary infiltrates; skin lesions; peripheral lymphadenopathy; ocular disease including iridocyclitis, keratoconjunctivitis, and chorioretinitis; hepatosplenomegaly; and neurologic, cardiac, and musculoskeletal involvement. Studies of patients with active sarcoidosis reveal immunologic abnormalities, features of which are cutaneous anergy and depressed cellular immunity with a hyperactive humoral system. A polyclonal elevation of immunoglobulins is found along with increased levels of circulating free light chains. Peripherally, excess suppressor T lymphocytes, excess B lymphocytes, and depressed numbers of T lymphocytes are characteristic. Sarcoidosis is characterized by spontaneous remissions; active disease usually responds to steroid therapy.

13. The answer is B. *(Fitzpatrick, ed 3. pp 520–528. Hanifer, Ann Allergy 52:386–393, 1984.)* Atopic dermatitis is a chronic inflammation of the skin characterized by pruritus accompanied by papules, lichenification, and eczematous lesions. There is typically a personal or family history of asthma, hay fever, or eczema and onset is usually in the childhood years. All patients have xerosis and are susceptible to pyogenic infections, especially those caused by *Staphylococcus aureus*, viral infections primarily due to herpes simplex and vaccinia, and superficial fungal infections. While IgE levels may be normal, they are typically elevated in patients with severe atopic dermatitis. Additionally, a defect in cell-mediated immunity exists and manifests as an increased susceptibility to cutaneous infections, a lower incidence of contact dermatitis from poison ivy, and a reduced rate of sensitization to dinitrochlorobenzene. The natural history of the disease is variable; 20 percent of patients will have persistent dermatitis that remains unchanged or worsens while the vast majority will improve. Complete remissions occur in 40 percent of patients by the end of the third decade. Treatment involves antihistamines for pruritus, antibiotics for secondary infections, and topical steroids.

14. The answer is B. *(Braunwald, ed 11. pp 1338–1340.)* The patient presented in the question probably has chronic active hepatitis, an autoimmune liver disease characterized by the chronic presence of anti–smooth muscle antibody and severe hypergammaglobulinemia. The disease usually is relentlessly progressive, developing eventual portal hypertension and episodes of bleeding. Antimitochondrial antibodies exist in 10 to 20 percent of affected patients but are more commonly associated with primary biliary cirrhosis. Chronic active hepatitis, which belongs to the lupus group of disorders, is infrequently associated with thyroid and gastric disorders. No consistent patterns relating HLA phenotypes and chronic active hepatitis have been found so far.

15. The answer is C. *(Braunwald, ed 11. p 333.)* The hyper-IgE syndrome (formerly known as Job's syndrome) is more common than was previously realized. Affecting both males and females, the syndrome consists of the development of severe atopic dermatitis associated with other atopic symptoms such as rhinitis and asthma. The most dramatic feature of the illness, however, is the sensitivity of patients to infections with staphylococcal organisms. Severe superficial and systemic staphylococcal abscesses occur, with osteomyelitis and pulmonary complications common. The condition is not familial. Some of the highest serum concentrations of IgE recorded in any disease have been associated with the hyper-IgE syndrome. It is common for patients to have IgE levels of 20,000 ng/ml. Intensive studies of leukocyte function in this disease have revealed two striking abnormalities. Polymorphonuclear cells fail to respond to normal chemotactic stimuli associated with staphylococcal infection and, in at least some patients, have a defect in those processes needed for the rapid uptake and initiation of the killing of staphylococci following phagocytosis. In addition there is a defect in immunoregulatory T cells that may be responsible for the hyperproduction of IgE by what appear to be normal B lymphocytes. Trials of levamisole, a powerful adjuvant, have been associated with too much toxicity and too little success to allow one to recommend this form of therapy. Currently patients must be maintained on prophylactic antibiotics when indicated, and it is necessary to make every effort to control the atopic dermatitis in the hope of preventing staphylococcal organisms from breaching the skin.

16. The answer is C (2, 4). *(Grieco, pp 92–99.)* Cryoglobulins are immunoglobulins that exhibit reversible precipitation in the cold. They may be *simple*, in which case they are of one immunoglobulin class, monoclonal, and almost always associated with multiple myeloma or macroglobulinemia; or *mixed*, in which case they are of more than one immunoglobulin class, either monoclonal or polyclonal, and usually found to be rheumatoid factor. While cryoglobulins occur in most normal people, they do so in low levels and are always polyclonal; pathologic cryoglobulins occur at concentrations of greater than 0.2 mg/ml. Associations include vasculitis, glomerulonephritis, collagen diseases, subacute bacterial endocarditis, syphilis, chronic HBV infection, and infectious mononucleosis. The finding of a monoclonal immunoglobulin should raise the possibility of an underlying lymphoproliferative or plasma cell disorder; IgM monoclonals are particularly associated with chronic lymphocytic leukemia (CLL), lymphoma, and angioblastic lymphadenopathy. Treatment is directed toward the underlying illness although plasmapheresis may be effective in the short term. Idiopathic mixed cryoglobulinemia may respond to cytotoxic drugs with amelioration of the associated nephritis, arthritis, and purpura.

17. The answer is C (2, 4). *(Braunwald, ed 11. p 1182.)* Berger's disease, the most common cause of recurrent hematuria of glomerular origin, usually affects young adult males. It is typically preceded by a viral illness. The hematuria may be gross or microscopic and the proteinuria is usually less than 3.5 g per day although the nephrotic syndrome is occasionally seen. Diagnosis is based on finding diffuse mesangial deposition of IgA usually accompanied by C3 and less frequently by IgG; Clq and C4 are not found. Fifty percent of patients have elevated levels of IgA, while serum complement levels remain normal. A poor prognosis is associated with azotemia, hypertension, and the nephrotic syndrome at the time of diagnosis and subepithelial and subendothelial deposits on renal biopsy. The disease generally progresses slowly and no form of therapy has been shown to be effective.

18. The answer is C (2, 4). *(Braunwald, ed 11. p 1480.)* Circulating immunoglobulins that can inactivate coagulation factors have been described in hemophiliacs, patients with systemic lupus erythematosus (SLE), elderly people of both sexes, and women immediately post partum. The antibody is usually IgG in nature, and in hemophilia the subclass IgG84 has been incriminated. The antibody can inactivate many factors, but antibodies to factors VIII and X are the most common. In conditions other than SLE, immunosuppressive therapy has failed to affect significantly the levels and functions of these antibodies. Such antibodies should be monitored routinely in the presence of SLE.

19. The answer is B (1, 3). *(Braunwald, ed 11. p 1774. Felig, ed 2. pp 548–549, 795.)* In general terms, glucocorticoids affect cellular processes, leukocyte distribution, and macrophages more than they affect humoral processes, leukocyte function, and polymorphonuclear leukocytes. Circulating lymphocytes, monocytes, and eosinophils are decreased secondary to redistribution of these cells into other compartments, while blood polymorphonuclear cells are increased. Within 2 hours of administration of steroids, there is a decrease in inflammatory cell accumulation at sites of injury. Lymphocyte proliferation, mediator production, autologous and allogenic mixed leukocyte reactions, and cutaneous delayed hypersensitivity are all suppressed. While there is no evidence that complement components are lowered, a small decrease in immunoglobulins secondary to decreased synthesis and increased catabolism is observed. Because precursor cells are steroid resistant, permanent damage to the immunological system does not occur. The cushingoid effects of glucocorticoid therapy can be minimized by administering the full 48-hr dose as a *single* dose of intermediate-acting steroid on the morning of every other day. However, this transition from daily to alternate-day administration should be attempted only after the manifestations of the disease are reasonably under control and is best made gradually.

20. The answer is E (all). *(Greenberger, Ann Allergy 56:444–448, 1986.) Aspergillus* is a ubiquitous fungus that is usually acquired by inhalation of its spores. While exposure is almost universal, disease is uncommon. Allergic bronchopulmonary aspergillosis is usually a complication of preexisting asthma and is characterized by transient pulmonary infiltrates, sputum and blood eosinophilia, elevated serum IgE, and an immediate-type skin-test response to *Aspergillus* antigen. Patients present complaining of fevers, chills, malaise, and a productive cough. If left untreated, bronchiectasis and pulmonary fibrosis are possible complications. Corticosteroids are the mainstay of therapy. Because evidence indicates that elevations in IgE occur prior to clinical exacerbations, prevention of acute flares is possible with prior use of steroids.

21. The answer is E (all). *(Braunwald, ed 11. pp 330–331.)* B lymphocytes are cells that mature in the bone marrow and have surface receptors that bind the Fc portion of IgG, some complement components, the Epstein-Barr virus, and, most importantly, specific antigen. The last is accomplished via a specific immunoglobulin receptor molecule. The cells have a short half-life (days) and are thus quite different from T cells that live for years. Oncogenic influence may cause these cells to proliferate and produce chronic lymphatic leukemia or lymphomas. B cells bind antigen and then divide to form plasma cells. The cells secrete an antibody product identical to that of the receptor on the B cell from which it was derived.

22. The answer is C (2, 4). *(Adams, ed 3. pp 707–708. Braunwald, ed 11. p 1996.)* There is evidence that the immune system is involved in the pathological processes that cause demyelination in the central nervous system and the clinical syndrome multiple sclerosis. It was observed more than 30 years ago that CSF immunoglobulin is increased in this disease. Although it must be stated that the cause of MS remains unknown, circumstantial evidence that an autoimmune process is important is very strong. The measurement of IgG in the CSF has proved to be a valuable diagnostic test. When the CSF IgG is elevated and the clinical presentation is compatible, a diagnosis of multiple sclerosis is likely. In recent years careful studies of the IgG found in the CSF of patients with MS have revealed that the IgG represents several oligoclonal peaks or bands superimposed on a background of polyclonal IgG. Plasma cells can easily be found within MS plaques, and the evidence strongly suggests that the IgG antibody is secreted locally. The significance of the oligoclonal bands is that, rather than all the B cells that circulate through the brain being stimulated randomly by an antigen or mitogen, selected clones of cells are being activated. This strongly suggests that either a limited number of brain antigens or infectious agents are producing the effect. Multiple sclerosis is not the only disease in which the CSF contains oligoclonal IgG. Many chronic central nervous system infections exhibit this finding. In subacute sclerosing panencephalitis (SSPE), chronic rubella, neurosyphilis, and cryptococcal meningitis such bands are common. Unlike the situation in SSPE, all attempts to absorb out the IgG from the CSF with viral antigens has been unsuccessful in MS. It nevertheless remains interesting that more than 50 percent of patients have B cells in their central nervous system making antibodies to measles virus. Many workers feel that the unbridled production of antibody, perhaps inappropriately, results from a lack of normal immunoregulatory T-cell activity. Suppressor T cells are drastically reduced in the blood of patients when an acute flare-up of their disease occurs. Not only the number, but also the function of immunoregulatory cells is disturbed in both the peripheral blood and the cerebrospinal fluid of patients with MS.

23. The answer is E (all). *(McCarty, Ann Allergy 55:421–433, 1985.)* Rheumatoid factor is an autoantibody directed against the Fc portion of IgG and is usually of the IgM class although IgA, IgG, and IgD rheumatoid factors exist. It is found in 60 to 90 percent of patients with rheumatoid arthritis although its presence in many other conditions reduces its specificity and its usefulness as a screening test for rheumatoid arthritis. Positivity increases with age. It is associated with rheumatic diseases such as scleroderma, SLE, and Sjögren's syndrome; viral conditions including mononucleosis, hepatitis, and influenza; parasitic infections; chronic inflammatory states such as tuberculosis, syphilis, and salmonellosis; neoplastic disorders; and chronic hyperglobulinemic states.

24. The answer is D (4). *(Braunwald, ed 11. pp 834–835.)* Desensitization of individuals who are hypersensitive to wasp and bee stings with whole-body Hymenoptera extract has been successful in some people, but the efficacy of this treatment in most cases has been subject to question. Recent investigations have shown that the major antigenic determinant responsible for anaphylactic reactions is contained within the venom of stinging wasps, hornets, and bees. Desensitization with venoms obtained from the specific species to which a given patient is allergic produces reliable and measurable results. Although it is true that only a relatively small number of deaths from hypersensitivity reactions is reported annually, these statistics have no bearing on an individual patient's situation. The danger for any given patient who has had an anaphylactoid reaction is very high. Many accidents occur annually when patients who know they are allergic to bee stings find themselves driving an automobile with a bee for a passenger. Patients should be taught how to use bee sting emergency kits containing epinephrine and should be counseled about the not-infrequent delayed reactions that occur after a sting. Reactions quite commonly occur after 24 hours and some reactions have been reported to start 48 hours after the stinging. Although desensitization with venom—as opposed to whole-body—extract is currently expensive, it is now the clear treatment of choice.

25–27. The answers are: 25-E, 26-A, 27-B. *(Braunwald, ed 11. pp 1389–1391. Murray, N Engl J Med 310:883–889, 1984.)* The biologically active chemicals secreted by activated lymphocytes are collectively known as lymphokines. More than 100 biologically distinct molecules have been described in the supernatants obtained from stimulated lymphocytes. Among these lymphokines is a particular type of interferon known as immune, or gamma, interferon. This molecule is of particular importance in the immunological cascade, for it exerts a potent influence on stimulating monocytes that have entered the tissues and matured to macrophages; stimulated by gamma interferon, their ability to kill intracellular pathogens is markedly enhanced. This includes the killing of cells infected with *Toxoplasma gondii*. T4 cells are a rich source of gamma interferon and, as these cells are a primary target in acquired immune deficiency syndrome (AIDS), it was perhaps not surprising that a study of the lymphokines secreted by the lymphocytes of patients with AIDS revealed a marked deficiency of many, including gamma interferon. This is of considerable clinical relevance as gamma interferon made by recombinant technology may be of considerable therapeutic benefit to patients with AIDS.

Sex-linked agammaglobulinemia is a disorder in which children are born without the ability to produce mature B lymphocytes. Lymphocytes that contain immunoglobulins within the cytoplasm can be found in the blood and bone marrow of these patients, but cells with immunoglobulin receptors on their surfaces are absent. Consequently, the cells of these patients are not able to interact with antigens and produce plasma cells that secrete immunoglobulins. A common associated abnormality is the absence of the first component of the classical pathway of complement C1q. At one time, it was thought that the absence of C1q might represent a second genetic defect in such patients. With the availability of intravenous gammaglobulin, however, replacement therapy for patients with this disease has improved, and it has been noted that after 6 months of therapy C1q is produced in these patients. This strongly suggests that C1q is not produced unless a stimulus is supplied by a normal concentration of IgG. This fact is clinically relevant because without the first component of complement the administration of IgG would have a limited therapeutic effect as complement would not be activated and the bactericidal activity of polymorphonuclear cells would remain defective.

One of the most common immunodeficiency states is known as transient hypogammaglobulinemia of infancy. In this defect young infants who should be able to make IgG antibody by the age of 3 months have a delay in the maturation of their humoral immune system. Most of these children can produce IgM normally but the production of IgG is delayed. As there is an obligatory maturational sequence involved in the production of the major classes of immunoglobulins in which IgM must be made before IgG, which in turn must be made before IgA, these children may suffer problems associated with a lack of tissue and mucous membrane protection. Most of these children spontaneously recover and produce antibodies normally by the age of 3 years. The defect in these children does not exist at the B-cell level; rather, there is a maturational delay in the ability of inducer T cells to supply those necessary maturation signals that switch immunoglobulin production from one class to another. The production of IgM for most antigens is relatively T cell–dependent, but the production of IgG and IgA demands T inducer cell function to be intact. If the IgG level falls below 200 mg/dl in these children, after maternal immunoglobulin delivered to the baby across the placenta has been fully degraded, the risk of severe infection becomes a serious possibility. Children with this problem most frequently present with diarrhea or recurrent upper respiratory tract infections and otitis media.

28–31. The answers are: 28-C, 29-C, 30-C, 31-C. *(Braunwald, ed 11. p 1425.)* Rheumatoid factor usually is an IgM antibody that has activity against aggregated or altered IgG, although rheumatoid factors of all immunoglobulin classes have been described. Juvenile rheumatoid arthritis, for instance, not uncommonly exhibits IgG rheumatoid factors that have antibody activity against aggregated or altered IgG. Rheumatoid factors are thus autoantibodies, and it seems certain that the macromolecular complexes so formed can activate complement mechanisms and cause joint damage. The activation of the complement cascade results in polymorphonuclear leukocyte infiltration into the joint fluid with subsequent damage to synovial tissues.

Though most frequently found in adult rheumatoid arthritis (90 percent), rheumatoid factors are also found in juvenile rheumatoid arthritis (25 percent), Sjögren's syndrome (75 percent), systemic lupus erythematosus (30 percent), and occasionally other inflammatory diseases, including leprosy and infectious mononucleosis. It is possible that an infectious agent generates an aggregated or altered antibody to that agent, and that this changed immunoglobulin stimulates the production of the rheumatoid factor in the susceptible person.

Rheumatoid arthritis can occur in agammaglobulinemic persons who by definition are incapable of making rheumatoid factors; it can also occur in a seronegative form in which no autoantibodies can be found. Usually such cases are milder than the seropositive cases of rheumatoid arthritis, but they raise the possibility that mechanisms other than the activation of complement by rheumatoid complexes may be important in the immunopathogenesis of rheumatoid arthritis.

32–36. The answers are: 32-B, 33-A, 34-B, 35-C, 36-C. *(Patel, Ann Allergy 50:144–149, 1984.)* Bullous pemphigoid is characterized by large, tense bullae that have a predilection for the inner thighs, flexor surfaces of the forearms, axillae, groin, and lower abdomen; mucous membranes may be involved, as well. Direct immunofluorescence reveals the presence of autoantibodies against the perilesional skin basement membrane zone in the lamina lucida where cleavage takes place. A mild vasculitis in lesional skin is also noted. While the disease is generally benign and self-limited, therapy with steroids, sometimes in combination with immunosuppressive drugs, is often used to control eruptions; relapses are infrequent. Healing generally takes place without scarring.

Pemphigus refers to a group of bullous diseases that includes pemphigus vulgaris, pemphigus vegitans, pemphigus foliaceus, and fogo selvagem. Pemphigus vulgaris is the most common type seen in North America and is characterized by acantholysis and the presence of IgG directed against cell surface antigenic determinants on keratinocytes. The bullae tend to spread on pressure (positive Nikolsky's sign) to involve large areas and heal poorly. Therapy involves corticosteroids along with steroid-sparing cytotoxic drugs. Recurrences are not infrequent and patients should be followed every 4 to 6 months after cessation of therapy for clinical or serologic recurrence of pemphigus.

37–41. The answers are: 37-C, 38-B, 39-B, 40-A, 41-D. *(Braunwald, ed 11. p 434. Hess, Transplant Proc 20:29–40, 1988.)* Cyclophosphamide is an alkylating agent frequently used for the treatment of lymphomas, breast cancer, lung cancer, and sarcomas as well as an immunomodulatory agent. Moderate doses of cyclophosphamide are preferentially cytotoxic to B lymphocytes as compared with T lymphocytes and therefore inhibit humoral immunity. While B cells are more sensitive to the effects of the drug than are mature suppressor T cells, they are slightly less sensitive than are precursors of suppressor T cells. At higher doses, helper T lymphocytes are also inhibited, thus leading to an immunosuppression of cytotoxic T-cell responses and an inhibition of interleukin-2 production. While the acute toxicity of cyclophosphamide consists of nausea and vomiting and anaphylactoid hypersensitivity, delayed toxicity entails bone marrow depression, hemorrhagic cystitis, alopecia, hyponatremia, leukemia, bladder cancer, and pulmonary fibrosis.

Cyclosporine is a fungal metabolite used as an immunosuppressive agent in organ transplantation and acts as a reversible inhibitor of T-lymphocyte function. Cyclosporine does not inhibit the cytotoxic activity of mature cytotoxic T-cells and has no effect on the differentiation or function of B lymphocytes. During drug therapy, interleukin-1, interleukin-2, and interleukin-3 are all inhibited; no effect on α-interferon or β-interferon is seen, but γ-interferon, a T-cell product, is markedly inhibited. While cyclophosphamide decreases both the number and function of macrophages and monocytes, no such effect is seen with cyclosporine, thus reducing the incidence of secondary infections. Of all the toxic effects of cyclosporine—hepatotoxicity, hirsutism, gingival hyperplasia, nephrotoxicity, tremor—only nephrotoxicity presents a major management problem.

Infectious Disease

DIRECTIONS: Each question below contains five suggested responses. Select the **one best** response to each question.

42. All the following statements concerning Rocky Mountain spotted fever are true EXCEPT

(A) fulminant cases leading to death in 5 days have been described
(B) the causative organism creates a vasculitis of small arteries and veins
(C) serum from affected patients agglutinates certain strains of *Proteus vulgaris*
(D) treatment with tetracycline will eradicate the organism
(E) patients recovering from the disease are resistant to reinfection

43. Medical personnel who have just completed cardiopulmonary resuscitation (CPR) on a patient with known meningococcemia should receive chemoprophylaxis with which of the following antibiotics?

(A) Penicillin
(B) Rifampin
(C) Sulfadiazine
(D) Erythromycin
(E) None of the above

44. A 35-year-old homosexual male presents to his physician with fever, lymphadenopathy, a maculopapular rash that spares the palms and soles, and hepatosplenomegaly. There is clinical evidence of encephalitis. The most likely causative organism is

(A) *Toxoplasma gondii*
(B) *Pneumocystis carinii*
(C) Cytomegalovirus
(D) *Coccidioides immitis*
(E) *Actinomyces israelii*

45. A 58-year-old man is being treated with penicillin for asymptomatic neurosyphilis. Which of the following is the best method of following response to treatment?

(A) Cerebrospinal Venereal Disease Research Laboratory (VDRL) reactivity
(B) The unabsorbed fluorescent treponemal antibody (FTA) test on cerebrospinal fluid
(C) Serum FTA test
(D) Cerebrospinal protein concentration
(E) Cerebrospinal cell count

46. Patients with cellular immune dysfunction are particularly susceptible to infection with all the following organisms EXCEPT

(A) cytomegalovirus
(B) *Haemophilus influenzae*
(C) *Mycobacterium tuberculosis*
(D) *Pneumocystis carinii*
(E) *Histoplasma capsulatum*

47. A fresh-water swimmer develops macules on his lower extremities 10 hours after bathing in an area known to harbor cercariae schistosomes. The natural history of the "swimmer's itch" includes

(A) the development of microscopic hematuria in about 2 months
(B) the development of a self-limited dermatitis
(C) the late development of cirrhosis and splenomegaly
(D) rapid abatement of fever after treatment with topical thiabendazole
(E) human-to-human transmission to persons in close physical contact

48. All the following statements concerning maculopapular rashes associated with infectious diseases are true EXCEPT

(A) *Mycoplasma* infections cause a maculopapular rash characterized by a prominent palmar or plantar involvement
(B) erythema infectiosum is associated with a confluent erythema over the cheeks and symmetric eruptions on the trunk, arms, and legs but rarely on the palms and soles
(C) echoviruses cause a maculopapular rash that may be associated with petechiae
(D) exanthem subitum (roseola infantum) produces a mild maculopapular rash that is largely asymptomatic even though it lasts 5 to 10 days
(E) maculopapular rashes are common in typhoid fever

49. Two days before the end of a 2-week vacation in the Caribbean, a 43-year-old man who had enjoyed good health experiences nausea, flatulence, epigastric discomfort, and watery diarrhea. Three weeks later, the diarrhea having persisted unabated, he consults his physician; the only abnormality found on stool examination is the presence of the trophozoite stages of *Giardia lamblia*. All the following statements concerning this patient's disorder are true EXCEPT that

(A) radiography may reveal irritability of the duodenal bulb
(B) it is important to check the stools of the patient's sexual partner for the same protozoan
(C) the significance of the stool finding is not clear; 3.8 percent of all stools examined in the United States reveal *Giardia lamblia*
(D) IgA deficiency, although commonly associated with *Giardia lamblia* infestation, is not likely to be a factor in this case
(E) rapid weight loss associated with the diarrhea would be consistent with a diagnosis of giardiasis

50. Chagas' disease exhibits all the following findings EXCEPT

(A) esophageal dilatation
(B) megacolon
(C) pancreatic pseudocysts
(D) unilateral conjunctivitis with edema of eyelids and face
(E) subacute myocarditis

51. Infection by *Plasmodium falciparum* is associated with all the following clinical signs or syndromes EXCEPT

(A) blackwater fever (hemoglobinuric fever)
(B) resistance to 4-aminoquinoline drugs such as chloroquine
(C) febrile episodes occurring every 72 hours
(D) cerebral malaria with coma
(E) high-density parasitemia

52. Rabies, an acute viral disease of the mammalian central nervous system, is transmitted by infective secretions, usually saliva. Which of the following statements about this disease is the most accurate?

(A) The disease is caused by a reovirus that elicits both complement-fixing and hemagglutinating antibodies useful in the diagnosis of the disease
(B) The incubation period is variable and, although 10 days is the most common elapsed time between infection and symptoms, some cases remain asymptomatic for 30 days
(C) Only 30 percent of infected patients will survive
(D) In the United States, the skunk and the bat have been the most important recent sources of human disease
(E) Wild animals that have bitten and are suspected of being rabid should be killed and their brains examined for virus particles by electron microscopy

53. A 60-year-old man had lived in Mexico for approximately 6 months. A year later he is seen for pyrexia, weight loss, and right upper quadrant pain. His oral cholecystogram is normal and liver function tests are mildly, but not diagnostically, abnormal. Which of the following would be the most useful diagnostic procedure?

(A) Serologic tests for amebiasis
(B) Examination of the stool for ova and parasites
(C) Examination of fluid aspirated from the liver
(D) A diagnostic trial of chloroquine
(E) A diagnostic trial of metronidazole

54. Appropriate specimens for attempted virus isolation or recognition differ with particular viruses. All the following viruses may be isolated from the sources specified EXCEPT

(A) echoviruses from stool or rectal swab
(B) rubella from urine
(C) varicella-zoster from vesicular fluid
(D) cytomegalovirus from throat swab
(E) arboviruses from cerebrospinal fluid

55. In a patient who has mitral valve insufficiency, prophylactic antibiotic treatment is recommended for all the following procedures EXCEPT

(A) cardiac catheterization
(B) prostatectomy
(C) cystoscopy
(D) sigmoidoscopy
(E) endoscopy

56. All the following statements concerning herpes simplex encephalitis are true EXCEPT that

(A) it is a common form of nonepidemic adult encephalitis in the United States
(B) the causative virus can usually be isolated from cerebrospinal fluid
(C) the cerebrospinal fluid in affected patients often contains red blood cells during acute illness
(D) it may result in necrosis of brain tissue and high fatality
(E) evidence of a localized brain lesion may be found on electroencephalography

DIRECTIONS: Each question below contains four suggested responses of which **one or more** is correct. Select

A	if	**1, 2, and 3**	are correct
B	if	**1 and 3**	are correct
C	if	**2 and 4**	are correct
D	if	**4**	is correct
E	if	**1, 2, 3, and 4**	are correct

57. A lifelong resident of Connecticut traveled to Arizona to work on a water project in the desert. Shortly after beginning work he developed fever, cough, and shortness of breath. He was diagnosed as having *Coccidioides immitis* by urine wet smear and culture. Other findings that he might be expected to develop include

(1) erythema nodosum
(2) arthralgias
(3) pneumonia
(4) a fleeting macular rash

58. Correct statements regarding herpes zoster (shingles) include which of the following?

(1) It probably results from reactivation of latent infection in persons who previously have had chickenpox
(2) It usually causes a bilateral skin eruption in a dermatomal distribution
(3) It is often associated with depression of delayed hypersensitivity by immunosuppressive chemotherapy
(4) Severe pain in an affected dermatome usually precedes the onset of the vesicular lesions and lasts until the skin manifestations clear

59. A patient with end-stage renal disease is maintained on chronic hemodialysis via a prosthetic subcutaneous arteriovenous fistula. Correct statements concerning infections of the conduit include that

(1) most are commonly caused by endogenous *Staphylococcus aureus*
(2) empirical antibiotic therapy should include coverage for *Pseudomonas aeruginosa*
(3) local findings of infection are absent in up to one-third of patients
(4) antibiotic therapy is curative in the vast majority of cases

SUMMARY OF DIRECTIONS

A	B	C	D	E
1,2,3	1,3	2,4	4	All are
only	only	only	only	correct

60. A 20-year-old man is admitted to the hospital; his chest x-rays are shown below. He is producing copious amounts of sputum and appears moderately ill; his oral temperature is 38.4°C (101°F). He reports that he has lost approximately 10 pounds in the past 2 months and complains of drenching night sweats during that period. Which of the following findings would be expected in this patient at this time?

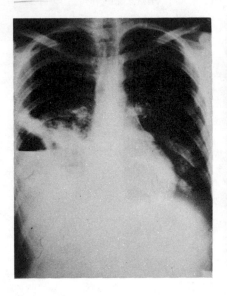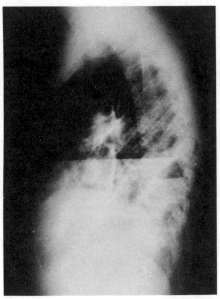

(1) Mixed gram-positive and gram-negative organisms in the sputum
(2) An absent gag reflex
(3) A history of drug abuse, alcohol abuse, or both
(4) A positive tuberculin test

61. Delta hepatitis may infect a person whose serum contains which of the following serologic markers?

(1) HBeAg
(2) Anti-HBc
(3) HBcAg
(4) Anti-HBs

62. A diabetic patient who requires insulin is seen in the emergency room with a painfully swollen eye, proptosis, and loss of external eye movements. She is acidotic; tenderness is elicited over the frontal sinus of the affected side. Rapid involvement of the other eye would suggest which of the following disorders?

(1) Osteomyelitis
(2) Orbital cellulitis
(3) Mucormycosis
(4) Cavernous sinus thrombosis

63. *Streptococcus (Diplococcus) pneumoniae* is responsible for a significant number of deaths. A vaccine containing capsular polysaccharides from the 14 pneumococcal types responsible for 80 percent of pneumococcal infections in the United States is available. Patients who should receive this vaccine include

(1) children who experience, in the first year of life, three attacks of otitis media caused by the pneumococcus
(2) patients with functional or anatomic asplenia
(3) patients with sickle cell disease who have not received a booster dose of vaccine for 2 years
(4) patients over 55 years of age who have chronic cardiovascular disease

64. A 28-year-old woman is brought to an emergency room with an infection in a foot wound sustained 7 days earlier. Examination reveals a moderate degree of cellulitis associated with the wound, diplopia, dysphonia, and weakness. Primary immunization at 4 years of age had consisted of three doses of tetanus toxoid and one booster 8 years later. She should now be treated with

(1) wound debridement
(2) trivalent botulinal antitoxin
(3) tetanus toxoid
(4) hyperimmune antitetanus gamma globulin

65. A 36-year-old woman has recently returned to the U.S. after a vacation in Egypt that included several swims in the Nile River. She has developed dysuria and hematuria; eggs of *Schistosoma haematobium* are found in her urine. Correct statements concerning this patient include that

(1) sexual partners are at risk of acquiring infection
(2) praziquantel is the drug of choice
(3) she should use separate toilet facilities until the infection has cleared
(4) if she is not treated, hydronephrosis may occur

SUMMARY OF DIRECTIONS

A	B	C	D	E
1,2,3 only	1,3 only	2,4 only	4 only	All are correct

66. A 37-year-old black man who works professionally with rabbits presents at his local emergency room. He had been well until 4 days earlier when he was scratched by a rabbit on his right hand. Within 24 hours an erythematous macule developed in that area. The macule rapidly became a large pruritic papule that is now ulcerated. He complains of fever (temperature 41°C [105.8°F]) and a very severe headache. He has a marked enlargement of the axillary lymph nodes under his right arm. Such a presentation is likely to

(1) require intensive treatment with streptomycin
(2) be followed by systemic disease with a severe oculoglandular infection causing serious conjunctival inflammation
(3) require a Foshay skin test for rapid diagnosis
(4) be caused by a gram-positive pleomorphic bacillus

67. *Histoplasma capsulatum* is associated with which of the following conditions?

(1) Pneumonia
(2) Pulmonary cavities
(3) Meningitis
(4) Febrile hepatosplenomegaly

68. True statements concerning antiviral therapy include which of the following?

(1) Vidarabine reduces the mortality of herpes simplex encephalitis
(2) Intravenous acyclovir reduces the frequency of recurrent genital herpes simplex infection
(3) Idoxuridine is effective therapy for herpes simplex keratitis
(4) Amantadine is effective in the prophylaxis of influenza A and influenza B

69. Cytomegalovirus is associated with which of the following?

(1) Hemolytic anemia
(2) Chorioretinitis
(3) Thrombocytopenic purpura
(4) Guillain-Barré syndrome

70. Antibiotics contraindicated during pregnancy include

(1) trimethoprim-sulfamethoxazole
(2) chloramphenicol
(3) erythromycin estolate
(4) tetracycline

DIRECTIONS: Each group of questions below consists of lettered headings followed by a set of numbered items. For each numbered item select the **one** lettered heading with which it is **most** closely associated. Each lettered heading may be used **once, more than once, or not at all.**

Questions 71–75

Match the following.

(A) Koplik's spots
(B) Agammaglobulinemia
(C) A vesicular and pustular eruption that begins when the patient is afebrile
(D) Acute cerebellar ataxia
(E) Pancreatitis

71. Mumps

72. Chickenpox

73. Smallpox

74. Echovirus

75. Measles

Questions 76–80

For each description of food poisoning that follows, select the microorganism with which it is most closely associated.

(A) *Clostridium perfringens*
(B) *Staphylococcus aureus*
(C) *Shigella sonnei*
(D) *Vibrio parahaemolyticus*
(E) *Yersinia enterocolitica*

76. Severe cramps, diarrhea, and occasional nausea and vomiting. Associated with cold or reheated cooked meats, gravy, or stews

77. Severe cramps, bloody diarrhea, and fever. Epidemics associated with contaminated water and food have been reported

78. Moderate to severe cramps, bloody diarrhea, and fever. Epidemics in the United States have been associated with ingestion of contaminated crabs

79. Severe nausea, vomiting, and occasional cramps and diarrhea. Associated with contaminated meats and dairy products

80. Severe abdominal pain and tenderness that may mimic appendicitis. Recent outbreaks in the United States have been associated with contaminated water

Questions 81–85

For each description of a patient that follows, select the figure or pair of figures (shown on this and the succeeding two pages) with which it is most likely to be associated.

81. A 40-year-old alcoholic man is admitted to the hospital with a 2-week history of fever, cough, and hemoptysis. Sputum culture is positive for *Staphylococcus aureus*. He is being treated with cephalothin but there is no response

82. A 20-year-old man afflicted with Hodgkin's disease is admitted to the hospital complaining of 5 days of increasingly severe vesicular rash and shortness of breath of 1 day's duration

83. A 58-year-old male outpatient has a 1-year history of cough and intermittent hemoptysis. Sputum cultures are positive for *Aspergillus fumigatus*

84. A 48-year-old man is seen in the outpatient department for evaluation of shortness of breath and wheezing. Sputum culture is positive for *A. fumigatus*. Skin and serologic tests for aspergillosis are positive as well

85. A 48-year-old woman who is receiving intensive treatment for thrombotic thrombocytopenic purpura is admitted to the hospital with fever, productive cough, and left-side weakness

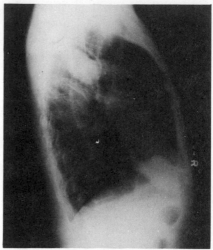

A₁

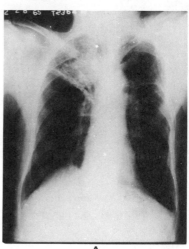

A₂

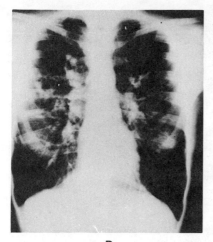

B₁

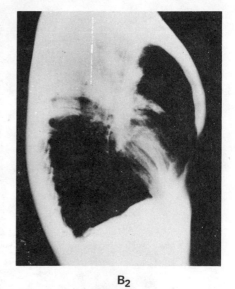

B₂

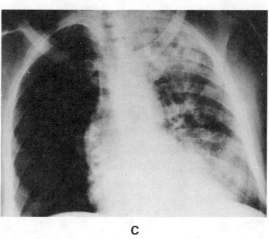

C

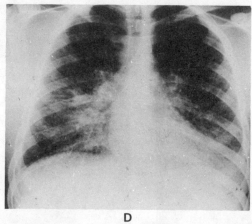

D

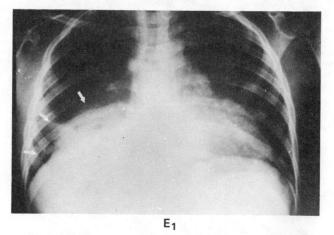

E₁

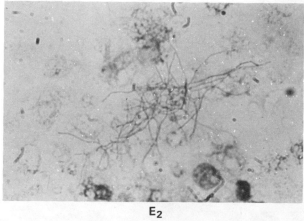

E₂

Questions 86–89

For infection by each of the following organisms, match the drug(s) of choice.

    (A) Metronidazole
    (B) Pyrimethamine and sulfadiazine
    (C) Pyrimethamine, sulfadiazine, and quinine
    (D) Sodium stibogluconate
    (E) None of the above

86. *Leishmania donovani*
87. *Entamoeba histolytica*
88. *Plasmodium falciparum*
89. *Toxoplasma gondii*

Questions 90–93

Match the following.

    (A) *Plasmodium vivax*
    (B) *Plasmodium malariae*
    (C) *Plasmodium falciparum*
    (D) *Plasmodium ovale*
    (E) *Babesia microti*

90. Central nervous system involvement

91. Paroxysms of fever every third day

92. Splenectomy

93. Blackwater fever

Questions 94–96

For each description below, select the drug combination with which it is most likely to be associated.

    (A) Chloramphenicol and phenytoin (Dilantin)
    (B) Isoniazid and rifampin
    (C) Tetracycline and antacids
    (D) Erythromycin and calcium supplements
    (E) Isoniazid and ethambutol

94. Decreased absorption of one drug due to the effect of the other

95. Increased risk of hepatotoxicity

96. Prolonged half-life of one drug due to a shared metabolic pathway with the other

Questions 97–101

For each description of a fungal infection below, select the microorganism with which it is most closely associated.

(A) *Blastomyces dermatitidis*
(B) *Histoplasma capsulatum*
(C) *Coccidioides immitis*
(D) *Aspergillus fumigatus*
(E) *Cryptococcus neoformans*

97. Disease occurs sporadically throughout the world. Susceptibility is increased by exogenous corticosteroids and in patients afflicted with lymphoma. Microorganism is isolated from pigeon droppings

98. Disease may be transmitted via fomites outside of endemic areas. Microorganism is isolated from soil especially around rodent burrows and is highly infectious

99. Disease associated with demolition of old buildings and excavations in endemic areas. Microorganism is isolated from soil high in organic content, especially bird droppings

100. Susceptibility to disease increases in patients who have quantitative or qualitative granulocyte defects or who are receiving corticosteroids. Saprophytic endobronchial—as well as invasive—infection occurs. Microorganism is isolated from decaying vegetation

101. Disease restricted to southeastern United States. Cutaneous, pulmonary, and disseminated forms may occur

Questions 102–106

For each pair of drugs below, select the type of drug interaction with which the pair is most likely to be associated.

(A) Enhanced anticoagulant effect
(B) Enhanced nephrotoxicity
(C) Increased incidence of thrombocytopenia
(D) Increased incidence of bone marrow suppression
(E) No significant toxicity

102. Tetracycline and dicumarol

103. Chloramphenicol and dicumarol

104. Azathioprine and allopurinol

105. Trimethoprim and thiazides

106. Carbenicillin and gentamicin

Questions 107–111

From the list of antimicrobial agents that follows, select the one that is the drug of choice for each of the diseases listed.

(A) Ticarcillin
(B) Spectinomycin
(C) Neomycin
(D) Vancomycin
(E) Sulfadiazine

107. Gonorrhea caused by penicillinase-producing strains

108. *Clostridium difficile*–associated enterocolitis

109. *Pseudomonas* infection in immunocompromised hosts

110. Nocardiosis

111. Nasal staphylococcal infection in chronic carriers

Questions 112–116

Match the infection-causing parasite below with the drug of choice.

(A) Niclosamide
(B) Mebendazole
(C) Thiabendazole
(D) Iodoquinol
(E) Quinacrine

112. *Strongyloides*

113. *Giardia*

114. *Diphyllobothrium latum*

115. *Ascaris*

116. *Dientamoeba fragilis*

Infectious Disease
Answers

42. The answer is D. *(Mandell, ed 2. pp 1082–1086.)* Rocky Mountain spotted fever is a disease transmitted by ticks and is the most common rickettsial infection in the U.S. More than 50 percent of cases occur in the South Atlantic region with a prevalence in the spring and summer. The infection is caused by the deposition of rickettsiae into the skin by ticks. A vasculitis of the small vessels is then produced, which may cause infarction in regions of the heart, brain, kidney, skin, and adrenal gland. Patients typically present with fever, chills, headache, and myalgias; a peripherally located, macular rash then appears on the third to fifth day of illness. While traditional laboratory tests are unremarkable, the Weil-Felix test, which relies on serum agglutination of various strains of *Proteus vulgaris*, is helpful in confirming the diagnosis. Therapy for 5 to 7 days with tetracycline or chloramphenicol, which are rickettsiostatic, is curative; resistance to reinfection follows recovery.

43. The answer is B. *(Braunwald, ed 11. p 576.)* Meningococci are gram-negative cocci or diplococci whose natural habitat is the nasopharynx; transmission from person to person is through inhalation of droplets of infected nasopharyngeal secretions. Meningococci may cause either epidemic or sporadic disease and the attack rate is highest for children between 6 months and 1 year. While some people harbor meningococci for years, nasopharyngeal infection is usually transient. Between epidemics, 2 to 15 percent of the people in urban centers carry meningococci in the nasopharynx. When sporadic cases occur, the carrier state in close contacts may approach 40 percent; during epidemics or in closed populations, the carrier state in close contacts may reach 100 percent. Because carriers, not patients, are the foci from which disease is spread, chemoprophylaxis should be administered to intimate contacts of sporadic cases of meningococcal disease. Rifampin in dosages of 600 mg every 12 hours for 2 days for adults and 5 to 10 mg/kg body weight every 12 hours for children will eradicate the carrier state temporarily and minimize the spread of meningococci.

44. The answer is A. *(Braunwald, ed 11. pp 791–797.)* Toxoplasmosis is caused by the obligate intracellular protozoan *Toxoplasma gondii*, a ubiquitous organism. The mechanism of infection is by ingestion of cysts or oocysts, transplacental transmission, blood transfusion, leukocyte transfusion, organ transplantation, or laboratory accident. Lymphadenopathy is the most common clinical presentation; when mesenteric or retroperitoneal nodes are involved, abdominal pain and fever may occur. In addition, confusion, stiff neck, myalgias, arthralgias, sore throat, urticaria, and hepatitis may be present. Even immunologically normal individuals may rarely present with pneumonitis, pericarditis, myocarditis, polymyositis, encephalitis, or meningoencephalitis; toxoplasmic encephalitis is a major cause of morbidity and mortality in patients with AIDS. *Toxoplasma* is estimated to cause 35 percent of cases of chorioretinitis in children and adults. The acute infection may be diagnosed by demonstration of characteristic lymph node histology, serologic tests, isolation from body fluids or blood, and demonstration of tachyzoites in histologic sections. Treatment is with pyrimethamine plus sulfadiazine or trisulfapyrimidines.

45. The answer is E. *(Braunwald, ed 11. p 649.)* The activity of neurosyphilis correlates best with cerebrospinal fluid pleocytosis; changes in the cerebrospinal fluid cell count provide the most sensitive index of response to treatment. An elevated cell count becomes normal in all cases within 2 to 4 years. To follow recovery, cerebrospinal fluid examination should be performed every 3 to 6 months for 3 years after treatment of asymptomatic neurosyphilis. The response of early syphilis to treatment should be determined by following the quantitative VDRL titer 1, 3, 6, and 12 months after treatment. The titer progressively declines and becomes negative in 75 percent of seropositive primary cases and 40 percent of secondary cases.

46. The answer is B. *(Mandell, ed 2. pp 1645–1647.)* Patients with Hodgkin's disease or AIDS or those receiving corticosteroid and cytotoxic agents all have in common a dysfunction of cellular immunity that leaves them particularly susceptible to infection with such pathogens as *Listeria monocytogenes*, Legionella, *Nocardia*, varicella-zoster virus, herpes simplex virus, *Toxoplasma gondii*, and *Strongyloides stercoralis*, as well as those listed in the question. Patients with humoral immune dysfunction, in contrast, lack opsonizing antibodies in their serum and therefore cannot adequately defend against encapsulated organisms such as *Haemophilus influenzae* and *Pneumococcus*. Granulocytopenic patients and those with defective leukocyte phagocytic activity are prone to infection with mycobacteria, *Listeria*, *Salmonella*, fungi, and certain viruses.

47. The answer is B. *(Braunwald, ed 11. pp 822–823. Hoeprich, ed 3. p 102.)* Human infection by the cercariae of one of the many nonhuman schistosomes is self-limited. On initial exposure, a mild dermatitis may not even be noticed. Sensitized persons develop more intense reactions, but the infection stops at this point without further progression. The disease is commonly found in Canada and the northern United States.

48. The answer is D. *(Braunwald, ed 11. pp 685–686.)* Enteroviruses such as echovirus can cause maculopapular rashes and occasionally papulovesicular or petechial rashes. Other viruses are capable of provoking erythema multiforme–like eruptions. The location of the rash provides a useful diagnostic criterion. Maculopapular rashes in which there is a relative sparing of the palms and soles are generally caused by viruses. Eruptions associated with drug reactions, bacteria, *Mycoplasma*, and *Rickettsia* often feature a prominent palmar and plantar eruption. The maculo-papular rash of roseola is usually transient, lasting only a few hours and rarely as long as 2 days.

49. The answer is C. *(Braunwald, ed 11. pp 800–801.)* Giardia lamblia is a pear-shaped multiflagellated protozoan that parasitizes the human small intestine. The organism is transmitted by the fecal-oral route. The infection is found worldwide, especially in regions of poor sanitation and personal hygiene. *Giardia lamblia* is diagnosed in 3.8 percent of examined stools in the United States and is the most frequently identified intestinal parasite. However, the finding of *Giardia lamblia* in the stool from the patient described in the question is highly significant. The orga-nisms frequently cause "traveler's diarrhea," characteristically beginning late in the course of the travels and persisting for several weeks. Giardiasis is commonly as-sociated with IgA deficiency, although IgA deficiency is not likely to be a factor in a previously well patient. Other conditions that predispose to giardiasis include gastrectomy and chronic pancreatitis. Irritability of the duodenal bulb often can be demonstrated radiographically. Rapid weight loss, along with lactase and disac-charidase deficiencies and general malabsorption, is commonly associated with giar-diasis. A study in New York demonstrated that all male "nontravelers" who had this infection were homosexual. Even in asymptomatic sexual partners of giardiasis victims, it is important that the infection be ruled out as a precaution against dis-semination of the disease.

50. The answer is C. *(Braunwald, ed 11. pp 787–790. Hoeprich, ed 3. pp 1193–1201.)* Chagas' disease, caused by protozoa of the genus *Trypanosoma*, involves the development of both megaesophagus and megacolon as a consequence of neuronal damage. The unilateral oculoglandular complex known as Romaña's sign and myocarditis are also well recognized features of the disease.

51. The answer is C. *(Braunwald, ed 11. pp 780–781. Hoeprich, ed 3. pp 1258–1259.)* The occurrence of fever every 72 hours is characteristic of early infection with *Plasmodium malariae*, or quartan malaria. This type of malaria can persist for many years with relapses as long as 20 years after infection. In falciparum malaria, however, a 48-hour cycle is seen.

52. The answer is D. *(Braunwald, ed 11. pp 712–715.)* Rabies is caused by a bullet-shaped rhabdovirus. The presence of neutralizing antibody to a knoblike pro-jection on the virus can be useful in diagnosis; a fourfold rise in the neutralizing antibody in serial serum samples is diagnostic in nonimmunized persons. In the United States, dogs seldom are rabid. The animals that represent the most danger are wild skunks and bats; raccoons and foxes also are possible carriers. The incubation period is variable, ranging from 10 days to 1 year with a mean of 1 to 2 months. In humans, only three definite recoveries from established infection have been reported. Nonimmunized animals that have bitten should be killed and their brains submitted for virus immunofluorescent antibody examination. A negative fluorescent test removes the need to treat the bite victim, either actively or passively.

53. The answer is D. *(Braunwald, ed 11. pp 773–778. Hoeprich, ed 3. pp 676–681.)* Amebiasis is prevalent in tropical and subtropical climates. Serologic tests, among them indirect hemagglutination, complement fixation, and agar gel diffusion, are positive in 80 to 100 percent of patients who have hepatic amebiasis. Response to chloroquine, measured by rapid decrease in both symptoms and abscess size, is the most important diagnostic test for this disorder. While metronidazole is an effective agent against trophozoites at all sites, a positive clinical response to it would not be diagnostic for amebic abscess because it also inhibits anaerobic bacteria. The classic anchovy-paste color associated with fluid aspirated from an abscess is by no means diagnostic of hepatic amebiasis.

54. The answer is D. *(Braunwald, ed 11. pp 665–666.)* Cytomegalovirus infection will produce a clinical syndrome indistinguishable from infectious mononucleosis. However, differential diagnosis can be made by isolating the virus from the urine and often from the buffy coat of blood. Rubella viruses are isolated from the throat and the urine, while arboviruses can be isolated only from the cerebrospinal fluid or a piece of brain tissue. Echoviruses may be isolated from the throat, cerebrospinal fluid, and vesicular fluid but rarely from the urine. Herpes zoster can be isolated from vesicular fluid and occasionally from the lungs and myocardium of infected persons.

55. The answer is A. *(Braunwald, ed 11. pp 531–533, 973–974. Hoeprich, ed 3. pp 242–244.)* Although no evidence exists that prophylactic antibiotic therapy prevents endocarditis, prophylaxis is recommended for all procedures that may generate bacteremias. Following cardiac catheterization, blood cultures obtained from a distal vein rarely are positive. Thus, prophylactic antibiosis is not currently recommended for cardiac catheterization. Bacteremia occurs commonly following other procedures such as endoscopy, cystoscopy, sigmoidoscopy, and prostate surgery.

56. The answer is B. *(Adams, ed 3. pp 558–560. Braunwald, ed 11. pp 694–695.)* In active cases of herpes simplex encephalitis, it is rare to culture herpesvirus from the cerebrospinal fluid. Once found, the virus is easily grown; a biopsy specimen from an affected part of the brain, procured early in the course of the disease, is the best means of isolating it. The isolation of the virus may in the future dictate therapy with an agent such as adenine arabinoside.

57. The answer is E (all). *(Braunwald, ed 11. pp 739–740.)* Coccidioides immitis has been found in certain semiarid and arid regions of Arizona, Texas, and New

Mexico, as well as in Mexico and some parts of Central and South America. Persons entering these regions from nonendemic areas are liable to become infected with this organism, which causes fever, malaise, dry cough, chest pain, night sweats, and anorexia. A macular or urticarial skin rash may be present within the first day or two of infection. Erythema nodosum or erythema multiforme and arthralgias may occur 3 days to 3 weeks after the onset of symptoms. The combination of erythema nodosum, arthralgias, and pneumonia represents the classic syndrome of valley fever (primary coccidioidomycosis). Headache and stiff neck occur much less commonly. Risk of dissemination from a pulmonary focus is very high in Filipinos and blacks.

58. The answer is B (1, 3). *(Braunwald, ed 11. pp 689–692. Hoeprich, ed 3. pp 886–890.)* Herpes zoster (shingles) usually is *unilateral* in distribution, causing a vesicular skin eruption that often halts abruptly at the midline of its dermatomal pattern. Despite a distinct association with Hodgkin's disease, zoster is not limited to patients with this disease. Nevertheless, attempts to define an underlying lympho-proliferative disorder are indicated because of this association. Frequently, pain along affected dermatomes persists for many weeks after the skin lesion has disappeared.

59. The answer is A (1, 2, 3). *(Mandell, ed 2. p 537.)* Prosthetic arteriovenous fistulas suffer an infection rate higher than that noted for native-vessel fistulas. Most infections are caused by endogenous *S. aureus*, although *P. aeruginosa* is also a frequent isolate. Infections may occur at the time of implantation or through needle punctures at the time of dialysis; bacteremia is an uncommon source but is not an uncommon complication. Local erythema, pain, abscess formation, and hemorrhage from disruption of suture lines may occur, but an absence of remarkable local findings occurs in up to one-third of cases. While antibiotic therapy alone may be sufficient for native-vessel arteriovenous fistulas, infected prostheses need to be removed.

60. The answer is B (1, 3). *(Braunwald, ed 11. pp 1080–1081.)* Primary lung abscess can occur at any age and is associated with the transient loss of the gag reflex, leading to aspiration. In the younger population, epilepsy and drug abuse are leading causes of loss of gag reflex. The average number of organisms cultured from transtracheal or transthoracic lung puncture aspirates is three. The organisms, a mixture of anaerobes and aerobes, are streptococci, *Fusobacterium*, and *Bacteroides* species. The significance of anaerobic organisms in expectorated sputum cannot be assessed since they are part of the normal flora. "Reinfection" tuberculosis, which also characteristically presents as a cavity, usually affects an upper lobe rather than a dependent pulmonary segment. Drenching night sweats can occur with many severe systemic infections besides tuberculosis. Successful medical treatment of primary lung abscess now can be achieved with a combination of antibiotics, therapeutic bronchoscopy, and vigorous pulmonary toilet. Penicillin continues to be the antibiotic of choice. In the penicillin-sensitive patient, either clindamycin or chloramphenicol is effective. Bronchopleural fistula and empyema may occur in association with lung abscess, as they did in the patient presented in the question; his x-rays can be observed to disclose an air-fluid level crossing the entire hemithorax. Drainage of the pleural space is mandatory in such cases.

61. The answer is A (1, 2, 3). *(Mandell, ed 2. pp 772–785.)* Delta hepatitis is an infectious disease of the liver caused by an agent first described in 1977. The virus contains an incomplete form of RNA and, unlike other viruses, requires the presence of HBsAg for replication. Infection with the delta agent, then, may occur with simultaneous infection with hepatitis B, as an acute infection on chronic type B hepatitis, or as a chronic infection superimposed on chronic type B hepatitis. The diagnosis can be confirmed only by liver biopsy as there are currently no commercially available tests for either delta antigen or antibody. The virus typically causes a severe form of hepatitis and may account for as many as one-third of cases of fulminant hepatitis. It is common in people with multiple parenteral exposures, but, unlike hepatitis B, it is uncommon in male homosexuals and dialysis patients. Because anti-HBs is the protective antibody in type B hepatitis, vaccination with immune globulin to prevent hepatitis B will also prevent delta hepatitis.

62. The answer is D (4). *(Braunwald, ed 11. pp 742, 1985.)* Patients who have cavernous sinus thrombosis with obstruction of the ophthalmic vein and involvement of cranial nerves III, IV, V, and VI are acutely ill and present characteristic eye findings of proptosis, chemosis, edema, and pain. Extension of the lesion through the intercavernous sinus to the contralateral sinus can be rapid. Although the commonest offending organism is *Staphylococcus aureus*, antibiotic therapy also should include coverage for *Proteus* and *Pseudomonas*. While mucormycosis and orbital cellulitis both enter the initial differential diagnosis of the patient discussed in the question, rapid spread of the lesion to the other eye in these disorders is uncommon.

63. The answer is C (2, 4). *(Braunwald, ed 11. p 528.)* The fatality rate in patients over the age of 12 with bacteremic pneumococcal pneumonia is 18 percent. The rate is significantly higher in patients who are over the age of 50, especially in patients with chronic disorders including cardiovascular disease, chronic bronchopulmonary and hepatic disease, diabetes, and renal insufficiency. The vaccine is recommended for all patients with sickle cell disease who are more than 2 years old. Unfortunately, the vaccine is of little use in children under the age of 2, who respond poorly to polysaccharide antigens, a circumstance that makes it difficult to protect them from many of the serious bacterial diseases that particularly affect this age group (e.g., *Haemophilus influenzae*, group B *Streptococcus, Meningococcus*). Severe Arthus' reactions can develop if the antigen is administered more frequently than every 3 years. The vaccine is 80 to 90 percent efficient in adults. Patients without normal splenic function are susceptible to overwhelming pneumococcal septicemia with disseminated intravascular coagulation. In such patients, the vaccine is particularly useful.

64. The answer is A (1, 2, 3). *(Braunwald, ed 11. pp 558–561.)* Clostridium *perfringens, C. tetani,* and *C. botulinum* all cause wound infections. *C. perfringens* may cause anaerobic cellulitis or myositis (gas gangrene). *C. tetani* and *C. botulinum* produce neurotoxins that have distinctive effects, but signs of local infection may be minimal. Tetanus toxin causes prolonged muscle spasms of flexor and extensor muscle groups. The masseter and respiratory muscles may be involved producing lockjaw and respiratory paralysis, respectively. *C. botulinum* toxin causes cranial nerve and symmetrical descending skeletal muscle paralysis; however, sensory function is not affected. Wound botulism is very rare; eight cases had been reported in the United States through January 1973. All clostridial wound infections require extensive debridement. For *C. tetani* and *C. botulinum* infections, antitoxin is given as well (preceded by skin testing for allergy since the antitoxin is produced in horses). Patients with any type of wound must be considered for tetanus prophylaxis. Adults are considered adequately immunized if they have completed a three-dose primary immunization series within 10 years, or if they have received such a series earlier and been given a booster within 10 years. Inadequately immunized patients should receive a booster if they completed the primary series, or a series of boosters if they did not. Hyperimmune antitetanus gamma globulin should be given only to patients who either have tetanus or have tetanus-prone wounds and have received either no previous immunization or only a single dose.

65. The answer is C (2, 4). *(Mandell, ed 2. pp 1573–1576.)* Schistosomes are endemic to Puerto Rico, Brazil, the Middle East, and the Philippines and require an appropriate snail intermediate host, which is absent in the U.S., for transmission. The patient in the question, then, is not a threat for spreading infection. Unlike *S. mansoni* and *S. japonicum*, which cause hepatomegaly and diarrhea, *S. haematobium* affects the ureters and bladder, where granulomatous reactions to the eggs occur and may lead to urinary obstruction. Praziquantel is a broad spectrum antihelminthic agent and is the drug of choice for all human schistosome species; it is well tolerated and only occasionally causes fever, headache, and abdominal discomfort. Other agents effective against schistosomes include metrifonate, which is effective against *S. haematobium*, and oxamniquine, which is effective against *S. mansoni*.

66. The answer is B (1, 3). *(Braunwald, ed 11. pp 613–615.)* It is most likely that this man is suffering from tularemia. This disease is usually contracted when *Francisella tularensis* organisms enter through a break in the skin. Rabbits frequently carry these organisms, and thus the disease is an occupational hazard for professional handlers of rabbit meat or pelts. The organism is present, however, in many other animals such as woodchucks, minks, muskrats, mice, rats, foxes, and squirrels. Body lice, snakes, and even fish have been thought to harbor the organism, which is a small gram-negative pleomorphic bacillus. It is extremely difficult to grow and requires expertise if the culture is not to be dangerous for laboratory workers. Included in the differential diagnosis for such a presentation would be plague, cat scratch fever, and sporotrichosis. Rarely the eye can be involved, but when this does happen a severe inflammation occurs on the conjunctiva associated with very noticeable lymphadenopathy in the preauricular and submandibular areas. Serology can help in the diagnosis of this disease, but antibodies do not appear until the end of the second week after infection and thus other methods are needed for a rapid diagnosis. The Foshay skin test employs specific antigens from the organism that will, in a nonimmunocompromised host, evoke a specific delayed hypersensitivity reaction by the end of the first week of illness. Of note, the white cell count is usually normal throughout. The recommended therapy involves the intramuscular administration of 1 to 2 g of streptomycin per day for 7 to 10 days. The serious nature of this illness, the widespread geographic distribution of the organism, and the many hosts that may carry the bacillus demand that physicians remain alert to the possibility of this disease.

67. The answer is E (all). *(Braunwald, ed 11. pp 738–739.) Histoplasma capsulatum* is an airborne microorganism causing primary infection of the lung. Lymphatic spread to regional lymph nodes and hematogenous spread to the liver and spleen are common. Infection in all these sites is suppressed by the immune response. A small number of affected patients may suffer relapse associated with hepatosplenomegaly and fever. This type of chronic disseminated histoplasmosis may be mistaken for a lymphoma. Disseminated infection may involve the adrenals, endocardium, pericardium, oropharynx, and larynx, as well as the meninges. Chronic pulmonary histoplasmosis resembles chronic pulmonary tuberculosis and may be associated with cavities.

68. The answer is B (1, 3). *(Mandell, ed 2. pp 270–281.)* Because viruses are obligate intracellular parasites, finding agents that specifically damage viruses and not the host cell has been difficult. There are currently several agents that are effective for a number of viral diseases. Acyclovir, an agent whose activity is limited to the herpes viruses, works by inhibiting viral DNA polymerase. It is particularly effective in primary genital herpes simplex infection in decreasing viral shedding, the duration of symptoms, and time to healing; the frequency of recurrent attacks, however, is not affected. It is successful in preventing and treating mucocutaneous herpes simplex infection in immunocompromised patients, as well. Acyclovir also has activity against herpes zoster infection in both immunocompetent and immunocompromised patients. Amantadine is effective only in the prevention and treatment of influenza A. It is generally well tolerated. Vidarabine is effective therapy for herpes simplex encephalitis, infections of herpes zoster in immunosuppressed patients, and in herpes simplex keratoconjunctivitis. Its mechanism of action is not known. Idoxuridine is also effective in herpes simplex conjunctivitis but is ineffective in herpes simplex encephalitis. Patients with allergic reactions to this agent may respond to therapy with vidarabine.

69. The answer is E (all). *(Mandell, ed 2. pp 960–969.)* Cytomegalovirus (CMV) is a human herpes virus whose transmission is through close interpersonal contact or by transfer of body fluids and tissues. In healthy adults, infection is usually subclinical or nonspecific, although a wide range of presentations may occur; meningoencephalitis, Guillain-Barré syndrome, hemolytic anemia, granulomatous hepatitis, and myocarditis are well described and usually seen as complications of CMV-induced mononucleosis. In the immunocompromised host, CMV infection still remains frequently asymptomatic, although fever, mononucleosis, hepatitis, and interstitial pneumonia are not uncommon manifestations. Congenital acquired infections are symptomatic in less than 25 percent of cases; when symptomatic, jaundice, microcephaly, motor disorders, and chorioretinitis are complications. Diagnosis is made through isolating the virus or by demonstrating a rise in antibody titers.

70. The answer is E (all). *(Chow, Rev Infect Dis 7:287–313, 1985.)* In terms of maternal toxicity, both erythromycin estolate and tetracycline are associated with hepatotoxicity, trimethoprim-sulfamethoxazole with vasculitis, and chloramphenicol with bone marrow aplasia. No known fetal damage occurs as a result of erythromycin estolate administration. In contrast, chloramphenicol is associated with the gray syndrome; tetracycline, because it avidly binds to developing bone, with inhibition of bone growth; and trimethoprim-sulfamethoxazole with various congenital anomalies. Essentially all antibiotics are excreted in breast milk, which is an important concern especially in relation to premature infants and those with hereditary enzyme defects.

71–75. The answers are: 71-E, 72-D, 73-C, 74-B, 75-A. *(Braunwald, ed 11. pp 682–683, 686–692, 703–706, 709–712.)* Although salivary adenitis is the most prominent feature of the communicable disease of viral-origin mumps, it is not uncommon to have involvement of the gonads, meninges, and pancreas. Males who develop mumps after the age of puberty have a 20 to 35 percent chance of developing a painful orchitis. Central nervous system involvement is common but usually mild, with 50 percent of cases having an increase in lymphocytes detectable in the CSF. Myocarditis, thrombocytopenic purpura, and polyarthritis may also occur as complications of this disease. An inflammatory change in the pancreas, however, is a potentially serious problem. Frequently, the symptoms consist of abdominal discomfort and a gastroenteritis-like illness. Fortunately, the complication tends to be self-limiting, but a number of cases of pancreatic insufficiency and brittle diabetes develop as a result of this infection. Liver complications occur in approximately 1 in every 200 cases.

   Although a polyneuritis and a transverse myelitis have been described, the most common manifestation of CNS infection with varicella is acute cerebellar ataxia.

While chickenpox is usually a benign illness, other complications such as myocarditis, iritis, nephritis, orchitis, and hepatitis keep up the pressure for the development of a vaccine. A live attenuated varicella-zoster viral vaccine is being tested in Japan, but no vaccine is available in the United States at this time.

It can be difficult to distinguish between the vesicular lesions of smallpox and chickenpox. Classically, however, a history of a rash with vesicles developing over a few hours would be typical of a chickenpox infection; vesiculation developing over a period of days is the rule in smallpox. While fever is characteristic of the prodrome of smallpox, it subsides prior to focal eruptions. Although not an entirely reliable criterion for differentiation, chickenpox lesions are seldom seen on the lower part of the forearms, whereas smallpox lesions are common at this site. Preparations of vesicular fluid under electron microscopy show characteristic brick-shaped particles with poxvirus.

One of the common complications for patients with sex-linked or acquired agammaglobulinemia is a central nervous system infection with an echovirus. This virus spreads via an extracellular route that makes it unusually vulnerable to neutralization by antibodies. In the absence of the ability to make a humoral response, this virus spreads rapidly and usually produces a fatal illness. Recently, the administration of intravenous preparations of gammaglobulin intraventricularly has controlled this serious complication of immune deficiency.

It may take from 9 to 11 days for the first symptoms of measles to develop after exposure. Malaise, irritability, and a high fever often associated with conjunctivitis with prominent tearing are common symptoms. This prodromal syndrome may last from 3 days to a week before the characteristic rash of measles develops. One or two days before the onset of the rash, characteristic Koplik's spots—small, red, irregular lesions with blue-white centers—may be visible on the mucous membranes and occasionally on the conjunctiva. Classically, the measles rash will begin on the forehead and spread downward and the Koplik's spots will rapidly resolve.

76–80. The answers are: 76-A, 77-C, 78-D, 79-B, 80-E. *(Braunwald, ed 11. pp 503–505, 599–601, 617–618.)* The most common causes of food-borne illness in the United States are *Clostridium perfringens* and *Staphylococcus aureus*. Both bacteria produce toxins in food during preparation. The clostridial food toxin is heat-labile, while the staphylococcal toxin is heat-stable. Fever is uncommon in illness caused by these toxins, which also is true of other toxin-mediated types of illness carried by food. Lower intestinal symptoms predominate with illness from *Clostridium*-contaminated food, whereas upper intestinal symptoms predominate with illness from staphylococcus-contaminated food.

Ingestion of bacteria with subsequent invasion of the intestinal mucosa has been associated with *Shigella sonnei* and other *Shigella* species, *Salmonella typhi, Vibrio parahaemolyticus,* and *Yersinia enterocolitica*. Illness caused by these microorganisms in food is generally associated with fever, abdominal pain, and diarrhea. Severe cramps and bloody diarrhea are associated with the *Shigella* infections. *Vibrio parahaemolyticus* has been associated with contaminated crabs caught in the Chesapeake Bay, and high salt concentrations in culture media are required to isolate this microorganism. *Yersinia enterocolitica,* which commonly causes infection in northern Europe, has recently been identified in the United States. Symptoms of infection with this organism may mimic appendicitis.

81–85. The answers are: 81-C, 82-D, 83-A, 84-B, 85-E. *(Braunwald, ed 11. pp 470, 627, 741–742, 1511–1512. Hoeprich, ed 3. pp 378–386.)* Acute tuberculous pneumonia (figure C appearing in the question) may occur when a large apical tuberculous cavity ruptures, spilling large numbers of organisms into the lower airways. The isolation of *Staphylococcus aureus* from the sputum is not, by itself, conclusive evidence of staphylococcal pneumonia. In most cases of tuberculous pneumonia, cultures and smears for *Mycobacterium tuberculosis* are positive.

Viral pneumonia (figure D) characteristically causes a diffuse pulmonary infiltrate. The coexistence of a vesicular skin rash may suggest the etiology. Varicella infection or herpes occurs with distressing frequency in victims of Hodgkin's disease and other lymphomas.

Aspergillus fumigatus may cause saprophytic endobronchial infection (mycetoma) in patients who have residual pulmonary cavities (figures A_1 and A_2). Characteristically, affected patients will have recurrent episodes of hemoptysis. The silhouette of the mycetoma (or fungus ball) may be seen in the cavity. Laminograms may be required to identify this type of infection.

Allergy to *A. fumigatus* may cause recurrent episodes of bronchospasm and eventually chronic obstructive lung disease (bronchopulmonary aspergillosis—figures B_1 and B_2).

Owing to its association with such diseases as systemic lupus erythematosus and polyarteritis nodosa (or to its treatment with high-dose corticosteroids), thrombotic thrombocytopenic purpura is conjectured to arise from a compromised host defense system. In patients afflicted with the disorders mentioned, opportunistic infections are likely. *Nocardia asteroides* may cause a necrotizing pulmonary infection with abscess formation (figure E_1). Signs or symptoms of an associated cerebral abscess may suggest the diagnosis. Although sputum cultures often are positive, a lung biopsy may be required to confirm the diagnosis (figure E_2).

86–89. The answers are: 86-D, 87-A, 88-C, 89-B. *(Hoeprich, ed 3. pp 674, 1133–1134, 1253, 1269–1280.)* Leishmaniasis is a zoonotic infection that involves rodents and canines and is transmitted when female sandflies ingest amastigotes while drawing blood from an infected animal. After a transformation in the insect's gut, the parasite is deposited on the skin of a new host at the next blood meal; humans acquire the disease when they break into this cycle. Transmission may also occur via blood transfusion, coitus, and contact inoculation. *Leishmania donovani* causes kala azar, whose onset may be insidious or abrupt and which may begin as a primary cutaneous lesion. Fever, diarrhea, cough, hepatosplenomegaly, and lymphadenopathy are manifestations. Pancytopenia, evidence of malabsorption due to extensive infiltration of the gastrointestinal tract, and circulating immune complexes are common laboratory abnormalities. Pentavalent antimonials, such as sodium stibogluconate, are effective therapy and relatively nontoxic.

Humans are the principle hosts for *Entamoeba histolytica*, an organism that causes infection of the large intestine. Diseases range from an asymptomatic carrier state to chronic mild diarrhea to fulminant dysentery; hepatic abscess, which may rupture into the lung, peritoneum, or pericardium, is the most common extraintestinal complication. Transmission is by the fecal-oral route. The diagnosis depends on finding the organism in stool or tissues. A large number of drugs are available for therapy: iodoquinol, diloxanide furoate, metronidazole, and chloroquine phosphate are several of the drugs available for the various manifestations of the disease.

Malaria, a protozoan disease characterized by fever, splenomegaly, anemia, and a chronic relapsing course, is transmitted to humans by *Anopheles* mosquitoes. After inoculation, the organisms invade hepatocytes, which rupture within 1 to 6 weeks, releasing the organisms back into the circulation where red blood cells are invaded. Falciparum malaria may have an insidious onset with fever, splenomegaly, headache, mental confusion, gastrointestinal symptoms, and edema as common manifestations. Cerebral malaria is an important complication in that it carries a mortality of 20 percent. Treatment with a combination of pyrimethamine, sulfadiazine, and quinine is curative in cases of chloroquine-resistant infection by *P. falciparum*.

Toxoplasmosis is caused by the obligate intracellular protozoan *Toxoplasma gondii*, which is transmitted by ingestion of cysts or oocysts or by transplacental transmission; infection may also be acquired by blood and granulocyte transfusion, organ transplantation, and laboratory accident. In immunocompetent patients, lymphadenopathy, fever, abdominal pain, stiff neck, myalgias, hepatosplenomegaly, and a maculopapular rash all may occur; in the immunocompromised patient, CNS involvement, in addition to the aforementioned manifestations, is commonly present. *Toxoplasma* is the cause of approximately 35 percent of cases of chorioretinitis. Treatment with pyrimethamine and sulfadiazine is curative.

90–93. The answers are: 90-C, 91-B, 92-E, 93-C. *(Braunwald, ed 11. pp 778–784.)* Although slow but definite progress is being made toward the development of a vaccine to prevent malaria, attempts in the third world to eradicate the *Anopheles* mosquito or its breeding grounds have failed. Malaria is on the increase throughout the tropics, and eradication attempts appear to have resulted in the survival of more hardy strains of plasmodia. In a number of areas they have become resistant to the simple antimalarial drugs. Nearly 2000 cases a year are diagnosed in the United States, mainly in patients who became infected while abroad. Of the four species of plasmodia that cause malaria, *P. falciparum* is the most important as it causes most of the clinical cases of malaria in the world and is associated with a large number of complications. Multiple infections of single red blood cells occur and organisms have the capacity to block the microcirculation in various organs. Cerebral involvement is common and frequently fatal in children. Seizures, focal disorders, delirium, and coma may occur. Blackwater fever occurs in association with malaria—particularly and perhaps only with falciparum malaria. For all forms of malaria the rupture of parasitized red cells with subsequent reinvasion of new cells is associated with paroxysms of chills and fever. Whereas *P. vivax* and *P. ovale* infections tend to cause alternate-day fevers, infections with *P. malariae* are associated with spiking every 72 hours (quartan malaria).

Babesiosis is a disease similar to malaria and also caused by a protozoan parasite that lives inside red blood cells. Babesiosis has been reported to be endemic on Nantucket Island but has also been found on other islands off the Massachusetts coast and in Georgia, California, Mexico, Yugoslavia, and Ireland. Although the disease can be mild, it is particularly serious in patients who have previously undergone splenectomy for an unrelated condition. In such patients very high fevers, drenching sweats, chills, lethargy, myalgias, arthralgias, and psychiatric disturbances are common. As many as 40 percent of the red cells may be infected. Recent studies would suggest that orally administered quinine in combination with clindamycin constitutes the treatment of choice for life-threatening disease.

94–96. The answers are: 94-C, 95-B, 96-A. *(Braunwald, ed 11. pp 349–350.)* Combinations of drugs may have unexpected effects. The gastrointestinal absorption of one of two combined drugs may be reduced, as occurs when digitalis and tetracycline are combined with neomycin and antacids, respectively.

Increased toxic effects from one or both drugs also may result from combined drug therapy, as in the following examples: rifampin with isoniazid (increased hepatotoxicity); aminoglycosides with skeletal muscle relaxants (respiratory paralysis) and, possibly, also with ethacrynic acid or furosemide (increased nephrotoxicity); rifampin with halothane (increased hepatotoxicity); and methoxyflurane with aminoglycosides or tetracycline (increased renal toxicity).

Finally, the half-life of one of the two drugs may be prolonged if they share a common metabolic pathway. In this manner, chloramphenicol prolongs the half-life of barbiturates, phenytoin (Dilantin), warfarin (Coumadin), and tolbutamide; isoniazid prolongs the half-life of phenytoin; and sulfonamides prolong the half-life of tolbutamide.

97–101. The answers are: 97-E, 98-C, 99-B, 100-D, 101-A. *(Braunwald, ed 11. pp 737–742. Hoeprich, ed 3. pp 451, 457–460, 479, 485, 1053–1054.)* Infections caused by *Cryptococcus neoformans, Histoplasma capsulatum, Coccidioides immitis, Aspergillus fumigatus,* and *Blastomyces dermatitidis* in some cases are known, and in others believed, to be transmitted by inhalation of airborne microorganisms or spores. Lymphatic spread to regional lymph nodes and hematogenous dissemination to extrapulmonary sites are common. The immune response in patients who have intact host defenses quickly suppresses or eradicates infection. But in patients who have lymphoma or are receiving corticosteroids, the pulmonary or extrapulmonary infection may be progressive.

C. neoformans has been isolated from pigeon droppings around the world. *C. immitis* is found in arid and semiarid regions of the southwestern United States and may be carried great distances by fomites.

H. capsulatum exists primarily in the Mississippi and Ohio River Valleys as well as in areas of West Virginia, Virginia, Pennsylvania, and Maryland; it is isolated from soil high in organic content, especially bird droppings. The spores may be stirred up by excavations or demolition.

A. fumigatus has been isolated from decaying vegetation around the world. Invasive infection occurs almost exclusively in compromised hosts. Saprophytic endobronchial infection may occur in patients who have bronchiectasis or pulmonary cavities. Hypersensitivity to *Aspergillus* may lead to episodes of wheezing and obstructive lung disease (bronchopulmonary aspergillosis).

The epidemiology and pathophysiology of *B. dermatitidis* infections are not fully understood. Cutaneous manifestations predominate but pulmonary, disseminated, and genital tract infections may occur as well.

102–106. The answers are: 102-A, 103-A, 104-D, 105-C, 106-E. *(Braunwald, ed 11. pp 349–350, 1472.)* The trend to the utilization of combination drugs makes it imperative that clinicians be conscious of possible interactions among them. One important interaction is the effect of some antibiotics on anticoagulants. For instance, broad-spectrum antibiotics, such as tetracycline, enhance the anticoagulant effect of dicumarol by decreasing the number of vitamin K–producing bacteria in the gut. Vitamin K is essential for the production by the liver of clotting factor II (prothrombin). Chloramphenicol causes an increase in the anticoagulant effect of dicumarol by interfering with the hepatic metabolism of the drug. In addition to the increased risk of bleeding during the course of an infection in a patient who is receiving both anticoagulant and antibiotic therapy, cessation of the antibiotic may be associated with an increased risk of clotting as the level of circulating anticoagulants is reduced. Many commonly used drugs, however, have the opposite effect of reducing the efficiency of oral anticoagulants. Such drugs include the barbiturates, digitoxin, quinidine, dexamethasone, and metyrapone.

Patients receiving the antibacterial agent trimethoprim in combination with the thiazide diuretics or furosemide may experience an increased incidence of thrombocytopenia. It is known that thiazide diuretics can act as myelosuppressive drugs, as can ethanol and estrogens. The sulfonamides, including trimethoprim, are suspected but not proven to produce immunologically mediated destruction of platelets.

The ability of allopurinol to effect partial inhibition of xanthine oxidase also makes this drug useful for the treatment of gout. It often is administered in situations, such as malignancies, in which rapid turnover of cells is associated with the release of large amounts of uric acid, thus incurring the risk of gouty symptoms. Allopurinol administered in combination with azathioprine (a 6-mercaptopurine derivative) can result in a life-threatening toxicity that produces bone marrow suppression. Aza-thioprine is normally converted to 6-mercaptopurine, an active metabolite, which is partially inactivated by the enzyme xanthine oxidase.

107–111. The answers are: 107-B, 108-D, 109-A, 110-E, 111-C. *(Braunwald, ed 11. pp 485–501.)* Spectinomycin is the drug of choice for the treatment of *Neisseria gonorrhoeae* genital infections when the organisms are producing peni-cillinase that would make them resistant to procaine penicillin. The drug is well tolerated, and a single 2-g dose injected intramuscularly is usually sufficient.

Chronic antibiotic administration may be associated with an overgrowth of *Clos-tridium difficile*. This organism produces a toxin that may cause an enterocolitis. Vancomycin is the drug of choice for its eradication.

One of the newer semisynthetic penicillins, ticarcillin, has pharmacokinetic properties very similar to those of the well-established carbenicillin but is three to four times as active against *Pseudomonas*. Excellent *Pseudomonas* activity can be obtained with doses that deliver much less sodium than would an equivalent dose of carbenicillin. Because of its great activity against *Pseudomonas*, ticarcillin is now thought to be the antibiotic of choice for immunocompromised hosts infected with this organism.

Nocardiosis is a dangerous intracellular bacterial infection that frequently in-vades the lungs and the central nervous system where large abscesses may form. The mortality with CNS involvement is very high. Sulfadiazine remains the treatment of choice because of its excellent activity against *Nocardia* and its ready penetration of the CNS. It is necessary to instruct patients to drink copious amounts of fluid when taking this drug if damaging crystals are to be prevented from forming in the urine.

Neomycin is no longer used parenterally but remains a valuable agent for steri-lizing the intestinal tract, and it is particularly useful when applied as a spray or an ointment for the eradication of staphylococcal organisms from the nasal passages of chronic carriers. A number of subjects who carry staphylococcal organisms in their nose suffer from repeated staphylococcal abscesses and can be a danger to family members who may not be carriers of the organism but whose skin may be colonized with organisms from the nose of the carrier.

112–116. The answers are: 112-C, 113-E, 114-A, 115-B, 116-D. *(Most, N Engl J Med 310:298–304, 1984.)* Primarily owing to travel abroad and an influx of refugees, parasitic infections in the U.S. have become an important consideration in recent years. Niclosamide is the drug of choice for the cestodes *D. latum, Taenia solium,* and *T. saginata.* While these cestodes usually cause asymptomatic infesta-tion of the gastrointestinal tract, immigrants from those regions where the worms are hyperendemic may have abdominal symptoms.

Ascaris infection is found primarily in the rural areas of the southern states and in immigrants from Indochina. A heavy worm load may lead to bowel obstruction, perforation, or biliary invasion. Treatment with 3 days of mebendazole is curative for this roundworm and for *Trichuris*.

Diagnosis of *Strongyloides* infection is particularly difficult and may require duodenal aspiration or biopsy. While the infection is usually asymptomatic, concomitant dysfunction in cellular immunity may allow the parasite to become invasive. Treatment with thiabendazole is curative.

Dientamoeba fragilis is an amoeba that causes diarrhea and is diagnosed by examining stained smears of stool samples. Treatment with tetracycline is as effective as treatment with iodoquinol.

Giardiasis is found throughout the U.S. and typically causes diarrhea, weight loss, and abdominal discomfort. Diagnosis is made by stool examination although duodenal aspiration or biopsy may be necessary. Treatment with quinacrine or metronidazole for 5 to 7 days is usually effective.

Rheumatology

DIRECTIONS: Each question below contains five suggested responses. Select the **one best** response to each question.

117. A 25-year-old man awakens with excruciating pain in the first metatarsophalangeal joint of his right foot. His physician identifies needle-shaped, negatively birefringent crystals in synovial fluid aspirated from the affected joint. The most desirable therapy for this patient would be

(A) allopurinol, 300 mg, and colchicine, 1.6 mg daily
(B) colchicine, 3 mg twice a day
(C) sulfinpyrazone, 400 mg daily
(D) indomethacin, 200 to 250 mg daily in divided doses
(E) salicylate, 3800 mg daily in divided doses

118. Ankylosing spondylitis is associated with all the following features EXCEPT

(A) peripheral arthritis
(B) abnormalities of cardiac conduction
(C) uveitis
(D) pulmonary fibrosis
(E) Sjögren's syndrome

119. Hypertrophic osteoarthropathy is associated with all the following conditions EXCEPT

(A) bronchogenic carcinoma
(B) osteoarthritis
(C) bronchiectasis
(D) inflammatory bowel disease
(E) biliary cirrhosis

120. A 25-year-old man who admits to frequent self-administration of intravenous drugs presents at an emergency room with a flat, nonspecific erythematous rash on his arms and trunks. He gives a 1-week history of pain and swelling in the fingers of both hands and a 2-day history of urticaria. He has a chronic cough but his chief complaint is of pain and swelling, of 24 hours duration, in his right knee. The pain is moderately severe with movement. The patient has a temperature of 37.8°C (100°F) and limitation of flexion at the metacarpophalangeal and proximal interphalangeal joints of both hands. A small effusion is noted in the right knee. The most likely diagnosis of this man's disorder would be

(A) gonococcal arthritis
(B) rheumatoid arthritis
(C) rheumatoid arthritis complicated by a septic arthritis
(D) tuberculous arthritis
(E) viral hepatitis complicated by arthritis

121. A 65-year-old woman who has a 12-year history of symmetrical polyarthritis is admitted to the hospital. Physical examination reveals splenomegaly, ulcerations over the anterior shins, and synovitis of the wrists, shoulders, and knees. Laboratory values demonstrate a white blood cell count of 2500/mm^3 and a rheumatoid factor titer of 1:4096. This patient's white blood cell differential count is likely to reveal

(A) pancytopenia
(B) lymphopenia
(C) granulocytopenia
(D) lymphocytosis
(E) basophilia

122. Arthritis of the temporomandibular joint may be caused by all the following diseases EXCEPT

(A) gout
(B) ankylosing spondylitis
(C) adult rheumatoid arthritis
(D) juvenile rheumatoid arthritis
(E) osteoarthritis

123. All the following statements about scleroderma are correct EXCEPT that

(A) skin telangiectasias are frequent and may be numerous
(B) weakness and atrophy of the proximal muscle groups may occur
(C) pulmonary interstitial fibrosis independent of pulmonary hypertension is common in advanced disease
(D) stricture of the large bowel secondary to fibrosis in the wall of the intestine may lead to intestinal obstruction
(E) the patient with CREST syndrome rarely has cardiac involvement

DIRECTIONS: Each question below contains four suggested responses of which **one or more** is correct. Select

A	if	**1, 2, and 3**	are correct
B	if	**1 and 3**	are correct
C	if	**2 and 4**	are correct
D	if	**4**	is correct
E	if	**1, 2, 3, and 4**	are correct

124. Correct statements about psoriatic arthritis include which of the following?

(1) Arthritis occurs in 20 to 25 percent of patients with psoriasis
(2) Ninety percent of patients with psoriatic arthritis, spondylitis, and sacroiliitis display the histocompatibility antigen B27
(3) Seventy percent of patients with psoriatic arthritis have seronegative symmetrical polyarthritis
(4) The flexor tendon sheaths in the fingers are often inflamed, producing "sausage" digits

125. Charcot's joints are associated with which of the following conditions?

(1) Syringomyelia
(2) Diabetes mellitus
(3) Syphilis
(4) Ankylosing spondylitis

126. Correct statements about the etiology and pathogenesis of degenerative joint disease include which of the following?

(1) Osteoarthritic cartilage undergoes increased metabolic activity and increased cell division, indicating that increased degradation and increased synthesis of cartilage matrix occur concurrently
(2) Degenerative disease of the wrists, elbows, and shoulders is relatively uncommon unless these joints are subjected to occupational trauma
(3) Extensive degenerative joint disease is found late in the course of acromegaly
(4) The routine laboratory tests show no abnormalities in degenerative joint disease

127. Correct statements about osteoarthritis include which of the following?

(1) It has an approximately equal incidence in men and women
(2) It is usually associated with osteoporosis
(3) It may be initiated by acute trauma to a joint
(4) It is usually associated with synovial fluid white blood cell counts greater than 10,000/mm^3

128. Relapsing polychondritis, a disease of unknown cause that leads to inflammation and destruction of cartilage, is characterized by which of the following clinical findings?

(1) The ears or nose may become swollen and tender
(2) Hearing loss may occur
(3) Hoarseness and recurrent pulmonary infections are common
(4) The disease is unresponsive to anti-inflammatory therapy

129. A 17-year-old white male high school student seeks medical advice because of recurrent low back pain and stiffness that last for a few days after each football game and extended practice session. The patient is otherwise healthy and has no family history of joint problems and no abnormal physical findings. Radiographic examination of his spine and sacroiliac joint reveals no abnormalities. Serologic studies are not helpful and the patient's erythrocyte sedimentation rate is 13 mm/hr (Westergren method). However, the patient is found to have the histocompatibility antigen HLA-B27 on his leukocytes. With this information, the physician can now advise the patient that

(1) it would be advisable to have an x-ray examination of his large bowel
(2) he should have an annual slitlamp examination of his eyes
(3) he should have phenylbutazone daily for the next year while his physician observes him closely for signs of developing spondylitis
(4) he has a 25 percent chance of developing significant spondylitis

130. Correct statements about Lyme disease include which of the following?

(1) The disease is caused by a spirochete that lives in the *Ixodes dammini* tick
(2) The disease has been found among patients with arthritis on both the east and west coasts of the United States and in Australia and Europe
(3) Tetracycline is the antibiotic of choice for newly diagnosed patients as it minimizes complications
(4) Lyme disease affects many body systems, and severe degrees of heart block may develop

131. Sjögren's syndrome is associated with which of the following diseases?

(1) Scleroderma
(2) Polymyositis
(3) Systemic lupus erythematosus
(4) Rheumatoid arthritis

132. The peripheral arthritis associated with inflammatory bowel disease is characterized by which of the following statements?

(1) It may be deforming
(2) It is associated with antinuclear antibody (ANA)
(3) It is more common in ulcerative colitis than in Crohn's disease
(4) It is often migratory

DIRECTIONS: Each group of questions below consists of lettered headings followed by a set of numbered items. For each numbered item select the **one** lettered heading with which it is **most** closely associated. Each lettered heading may be used **once, more than once, or not at all.**

Questions 133–137

For each set of synovial fluid data below, select the disease with which it is most likely to be associated.

(A) Degenerative joint disease
(B) Pseudogout
(C) Systemic lupus erythematosus
(D) Reiter's syndrome
(E) Rheumatoid arthritis

	Mucin Clot	Fibrin Clot	Appear-ance	Total WBC (per mm³)	Percent Polys	Synovial Fluid Com-plement	Glucose, Percent of Blood Level
133.	Poor	Large	Turbid	35,000	80	Normal	90
134.	Good	Small	Slightly turbid	1,100	15	Normal	98
135.	Poor	Large	Turbid	50,000	70	Decreased	75
136.	Good	Large	Straw-colored	10,000	25	Decreased	75
137.	Fair	Large	Turbid	50,000	55	Increased	75

Questions 138–142

For each condition select the drug with which it is associated.

(A) Indomethacin (Indocin)
(B) Gold
(C) Penicillamine
(D) Chloroquine
(E) None of the above

138. Interstitial nephritis

139. Goodpasture's syndrome

140. Blindness

141. Membranous glomerulopathy

142. Stomatitis

DIRECTIONS: Each group of questions below consists of four lettered headings followed by a set of numbered items. For each numbered item select

A	if the item is associated with	(A) **only**
B	if the item is associated with	(B) **only**
C	if the item is associated with	**both** (A) and (B)
D	if the item is associated with	**neither** (A) nor (B)

Each lettered heading may be used **once, more than once, or not at all.**

Questions 143–147

(A) Gonococcal arthritis
(B) Reiter's syndrome
(C) Both
(D) Neither

143. Uveitis

144. Balanitis

145. Arthritis involving predominantly joints of the upper extremities

146. Ten percent of patients HLA-B27-positive

147. Stomatitis

Rheumatology
Answers

117. The answer is D. *(Braunwald, ed 11. pp 1623–1631.)* Appropriate therapy of acute gouty arthritis can be divided into two phases. In the first phase, the acute gouty inflammation is controlled by anti-inflammatory agents administered, usually, in conjunction with an analgesic agent in severe cases. In the second phase, the serum rate level is lowered by uricosuric agents or drugs designed to inhibit the development of uric acid. Traditionally, acute gouty inflammation has been controlled by giving colchicine on an hourly basis until a therapeutic response occurs. However, as many as 80 percent of gout patients cannot achieve satisfactory therapeutic levels with colchicine because of the toxicity of the drug. Recently, anti-inflammatory drugs such as indomethacin or phenylbutazone have been found to be equally as effective as colchicine and to have fewer of the gastrointestinal side effects frequently associated with colchicine. Allopurinol, a xanthine oxidase inhibitor, and the uricosuric agents probenecid and sulfinpyrazone effectively reverse hyperuricemia, but do not relieve inflammation associated with acute attacks of gouty arthritis. The intense pain of gout may well require an initial dose of a narcotic analgesic to make the patient more comfortable while the anti-inflammatory agents have time to suppress the arthritis.

118. The answer is E. *(Braunwald, ed 11. pp 1434–1436.)* Ankylosing spondylitis, an arthritis of the joints of the spine, also involves the hip, shoulder, and, in 25 percent of patients, the peripheral joints. It is characteristically associated with aortic regurgitation, conduction abnormalities that may require pacemaker therapy, acute anterior uveitis in 30 percent of patients, and, in long-standing disease, bilateral pulmonary fibrosis of the upper lobe. HLA-B27 is found in the vast majority of patients. Ankylosing spondylitis must be differentiated from other diseases associated with spondylitis, such as inflammatory bowel disease, psoriatic arthritis, and Reiter's syndrome. The clinical course is characterized by remissions and exacerbations, although a persistently progressive course may occur. Symptomatic relief may be achieved using either salicylates or any of the nonsteroidal anti-inflammatory drugs. The uveitis is treated with intraocular steroids. The progression of the disease is not halted, however, by any of these measures.

119. The answer is B. *(Braunwald, ed 11. p 1466.)* Hypertrophic osteoarthropathy, commonly associated with primary intrathoracic malignancies, is characterized by periosteal thickening and new bone formation over the distal ends of bones. It is usually seen with clubbing and may cause an arthritis of the fingers, wrists, knees, and ankles. Patients usually complain of mild arthralgias and a burning sensation of the hands and feet. Symptoms are usually controlled with anti-inflammatory agents and the condition may disappear with resolution of the underlying disease. Hypertrophic osteoarthropathy is also associated with intrathoracic chronic infections such as lung abscess, bronchiectasis, and empyema; with cyanotic congenital heart disease; with predominantly diarrheal states such as inflammatory bowel disease, intestinal tuberculosis, sprue, and amebic or bacillary dysentery.

120. The answer is E. *(Braunwald, ed 11. pp 1462–1465.)* Arthritis is a relatively common manifestation of type B hepatitis, as is the occurrence of urticaria in the prodromal phase. Clinically detectable jaundice may not develop for a few days or even weeks after the onset of a severe arthritis, which tends to be migratory and involves both small and large joints. As the involvement in the hands is frequently symmetrical, it is easily confused with rheumatoid arthritis. The arthritis may be accompanied by a rash. Suspicion of a hepatitis-induced arthritis will be confirmed by the detection of abnormal liver functions, especially elevated liver enzymes, while Australia antigen, and perhaps antibody, will be detected in the serum and joint fluid in which complement levels may also be low, indicating active antigen-antibody complex deposition. Permanent joint damage may develop rapidly as a complication of septic arthritis. Early diagnosis with appropriate management of the arthritis is essential if this complication is to be avoided. Infectious arthritis can arise from viral, bacterial, and mycotic infections and although the diagnosis relies heavily on examination and culture of the joint fluid, these observations may not be immediately helpful. *Haemophilus influenzae,* which frequently causes meningitis in children, is most often responsible for a septic arthritis in this age group. Septic arthritis due to *Staphylococcus aureus* is now frequently encountered in drug-addicted persons who administer their drugs by an intravenous route. Gonococcal arthritis remains a disease of sexually active persons, usually women, who are particularly prone to develop a bacteremia at the time of menstruation. Bilateral and symmetrical synovial thickening of the joints of the hands and wrists is unusual in gonococcal arthritis, although skin rashes are common. Rheumatoid arthritis is more common in women than men but usually is not associated with a rash, although Still's disease occurring in adults features a generalized rash. Patients with rheumatoid arthritis who present with sudden localized pain and swelling should be carefully evaluated for a septic joint; underlying joint disease increases susceptibility to secondary septic involvement of a joint space. Bacterial sepsis usually presents with severe splinting and restriction of movement. Tuberculous arthritis, although now very rare, is more likely to arise in children than adults. Arthritis and inflammation around the infected joints develop slowly, with spine, hips, and knees being particularly susceptible. Symmetrical disease of the hands is rare in tuberculosis, while the thickened synovium found in this condition has a characteristic boggy or doughy feeling.

121. The answer is C. *(Braunwald, ed 11. pp 1424–1425.)* Felty's syndrome consists of a triad of rheumatoid arthritis, splenomegaly, and leukopenia. In contrast with the lymphopenia observed in patients who have systemic lupus erythematosus, the leukopenia of Felty's syndrome is related to a reduction in the number of circulating polymorphonuclear leukocytes. The mechanism of the granulocytopenia is poorly understood. Felty's syndrome tends to occur in people who have had active rheumatoid arthritis for a prolonged period. These patients commonly have other systemic features of rheumatoid disease such as nodules, skin ulcerations, the sicca complex, peripheral sensory and motor neuropathy, and arteritic lesions.

122. The answer is A. *(Braunwald, ed 11. p 168.)* Temporomandibular joint involvement is a classic feature of juvenile rheumatoid arthritis and, when present prior to closure of the epiphysis of the mandible, results in micrognathia. Adult rheumatoid arthritis frequently causes temporomandibular joint symptoms, and osteoarthritis and ankylosing spondylitis affect the joint in a smaller percentage of cases. Gout does not affect this particular joint.

123. The answer is D. *(Braunwald, ed 11. pp 1428–1432.)* Scleroderma, or progressive systemic sclerosis, is a disease in which many organs may be damaged by the relentless deposition of fibrous connective tissue. Most frequently affected are the skin and blood vessels, but the gastrointestinal tract, lungs, kidneys, and heart are also commonly involved. Although scleroderma that is localized to the skin may be compatible with a normal life span, systemic involvement is often fatal. Gradual thickening of the skin is associated with loss of mobility that will eventually make it difficult to flex the finger joints normally. In addition and classically, telangiectasias are prominent. When muscles are involved in the sclerodermatous destructive process they are usually proximal muscle groups, especially around the shoulder and girdle, that are involved in a polymyositis-like syndrome. There has been much recent interest in the lung disease that commonly complicates the course of scleroderma. Pulmonary hypertension is common and may lead to cor pulmonale when pulmonary blood vessels are affected by the fibrotic process. However, interstitial pulmonary fibrosis can develop with alveolar involvement. Although this may represent the direct effects of the disease process, esophageal reflux is so common that a number of studies have demonstrated fibrotic changes in the lung secondary to the aspiration of gastric contents, particularly while the patient sleeps at night. In such cases surgical intervention may be necessary to protect the lungs. As fibrosis destroys the autonomic nerve supply to the intestinal tract, hypomotility and dilatation of the intestinal tract occur. Slowing of the passage of food content through the intestinal tract may lead to a malabsorption syndrome. The CREST variant of scleroderma involves the deposition of *c*alcium in the skin, the presence of *R*aynaud's phenomenon, *e*sophageal hypomotility, *s*clerodactyly, and *t*elangiectasis. It is of interest that while extensive myocardial dysfunction can occur secondary to fibrotic changes in the heart, this is extremely unusual in the CREST variety of scleroderma. Serological evidence would suggest a different immunologic mechanism may be responsible for the CREST syndrome. Three forms of antinuclear antibody appear to be specific for scleroderma. Antibody to Scl-70 antigen as well as to the nuclear centromere and nucleolar antigens has been demonstrated. The anticentromere antibody is primarily seen in patients with the CREST form of the disease. Treatment of the disease is mainly symptomatic. Steroids do not help, but the malabsorption syndrome is frequently helped by the use of broad spectrum antibiotics. Captopril, the oral angiotensin-converting enzyme inhibitor, has helped a number of patients with serious hypertension, and in severe ischemic crises sympathectomy has reversed some of the effects of the Raynaud's phenomenon.

124. The answer is C (2, 4). *(Braunwald, ed 11. pp 1460–1461.)* Five percent of patients suffering from psoriasis develop one of a number of arthritic syndromes. Usually the psoriasis is present for many years before joint inflammation develops, but occasionally the opposite can be seen. The different syndromes associated with psoriatic arthritis are subgrouped according to the joints involved. At least 70 percent of patients with psoriatic arthritis have a monoarticular or asymmetrical oligoarticular arthritis. The smaller joints in the hands and feet can be involved and a classic finding is the sausage-shaped digits produced when the flexor tendon sheaths in the fingers become swollen and inflamed. Fifteen percent of patients with psoriatic arthritis present with a seronegative rheumatoid arthritis–type picture. Occasionally the arthritis is seropositive; because both psoriasis and rheumatoid arthritis are common diseases, it is likely that this represents two diseases occurring simultaneously. A third group of patients suffer from arthritis that is limited to the distal interphalangeal joints, and with this form the destructive pitting of the fingernails that is a characteristic of this disease is most noticeable. A rare form of psoriatic arthritis is associated with a destructive arthropathy. This form tends to occur in men more than women, although psoriatic arthritis in general is more common in females. A strong link to the spondyloarthritides in general is obvious from the fact that 90 percent of patients with psoriatic arthritis, spondylitis, and sacroiliitis display the histocompatibility antigen B27 that is so strongly associated with ankylosing spondylitis. Between 10 and 20 percent of patients with psoriatic arthritis have hyperuricemia, but this rarely leads to crystal formation in joints and is more a reflection of the severity of the skin disease. The treatment of this form of arthritis is similar to that of rheumatoid arthritis.

125. The answer is A (1, 2, 3). *(Braunwald, ed 11. p 1465.)* Charcot's joints occur in those conditions that are characterized by abnormalities of proprioception and deep pain sensation. A single joint is involved initially and other joints follow, the distribution being determined by the underlying disorder. In tabes dorsalis, the knees, hips, ankles, and lumbar spine are involved; in diabetes, the tarsometatarsal, metatarsophalangeal, and tarsal joints are affected; and in syringomyelia, the shoulders, elbows, and cervical spine reveal pathologic changes. The involved joints suffer recurrent fractures with secondary overgrowth of bone. Effusions, pain, and joint instability are the end results. Braces and treatment of the underlying disorder are the only effective therapies.

126. The answer is E (all). *(Braunwald, ed 11. pp 1456–1458.)* The major characteristics of degenerative joint disease are loss of joint cartilage and hypertrophy of bone. Within osteoarthritic cartilage, there is a marked increase in metabolic activity owing to the increased rate of destruction of cartilage accompanied by an increased synthesis of cartilage matrix. The increased proteolytic activity in the joint space is associated with higher than normal levels of proteases, particularly cathepsin D and similar hydrolases. As the disease progresses, cartilage is steadily lost from the joint because anabolic processes are unable to keep up with catabolism. Chronic occupational trauma to joints—such as that encountered by air hammer workers—may result in osteoarthritis occurring in joints that usually are not involved in this disease, such as the wrists, elbows, and shoulders. The excessive secretion of growth hormone in patients with acromegaly is thought to be responsible for the thickening of synovial tissues and the overgrowth of joint cartilage that characterize the articular changes seen early in this disease. If acromegaly is untreated, marked degenerative changes will occur in joints. Because routine laboratory tests cannot detect the abnormalities, radiologic observation of changes occurring in joints still provides the most useful information for arriving at a diagnosis of degenerative joint disease.

127. The answer is B (1, 3). *(Braunwald, ed 11. pp 1456–1458.)* Osteoarthritis is the most common form of joint disease in adults. When all age groups are considered, men and women are equally affected. The pathologic process is characterized by deterioration of articular cartilage and remodeling of subchondral bone to produce the characteristic picture of joint space narrowing, subchondral eburnation, and osteophyte formation. Joint trauma may initiate this disease even in young people.

128. The answer is A (1, 2, 3). *(Braunwald, ed 11. pp 1465–1466.)* While it is suspected that metabolic defects, immunological defects, or both produce the chronic inflammation that results in the relapsing polychondritis syndrome, the pathogenesis of the disease remains unclear. The characteristic basophilic staining of normal cartilage that is revealed in hematoxylin and eosin preparations is lost in this disease. Inflammation in the cartilage of the nose and ears, which occurs in at least 80 percent of affected patients, produces the classic clinical signs of this condition. Both the ears and the nose become inflamed and painful, and progressive destruction of cartilage frequently results in severe disfigurement of the nose and drooping of the ears. The cartilaginous components of the external auditory meatus may be affected and progressive destruction may lead to a severe impairment of hearing. When relapsing polychondritis affects the upper respiratory tract and the bronchi, hoarseness may develop from involvement of the larynx. Reports have documented the fact that severe tracheal stenosis and even death from suffocation may occur if this major airway is destroyed. Recurrent pulmonary infections follow collapse of the cartilaginous tissue in the bronchi, leading to obstruction and stasis and subsequent bacterial overgrowth. The usual time of onset of this disease is in middle age and its natural history is characterized by periods of remission. Fortunately, the inflammation is sensitive to moderate doses of corticosteroids, which afford considerable relief for affected patients.

129. The answer is D (4). *(Braunwald, ed 11. pp 1434–1436.)* The histocompatibility antigen HLA-B27 is the histocompatibility protein complex that represents the expression of the HLA-B27 allele situated at the B locus on the short arm of chromosome 6. This location is very close to the D locus of chromosome 6, which, apart from being responsible for the expression of D locus antigens on the surface of many cells, especially B cells and macrophages, is thought to be intimately associated with the various alleles that determine the appropriateness and efficiency of immunoregulatory function at the level of the T cell. When alleles of different loci are associated in the population more frequently than would be expected by chance, the phenomenon is termed linkage disequilibrium. HLA-B27 antigens are associated with ankylosing spondylitis because the HLA-B27 allele is associated by linkage disequilibrium with alleles near the D locus that failed to prevent the development of an inflammatory reaction in certain tissues such as the uveal tract of the eye, the vertebral column, joint spaces, and the urethral tract. The inflammation in these tissues is most commonly ascribed to defects in immunoregulation. Although 90 percent of patients with ankylosing spondylitis have the HLA-B27 gene, as opposed to 7 percent of the normal white population, the presence of the gene in the absence of a family history and convincing manifestation of this disorder indicates a risk no greater than 25 percent for developing spondylitis. Only 20 to 30 percent of patients with definite spondylitis develop uveitis. Thus, routine examination of the eye in asymptomatic patients is not warranted. The HLA-B27 gene is found in 60 to 75 percent of patients with enteropathic spondylitis. However, the presence of the gene product per se is insufficient reason to examine the large bowel. The most likely diagnosis in the patient presented in the question is local traumatic injury associated with his athletic endeavors. Phenylbutazone, which can be effective in spondylitis, has side effects and is not recommended in the absence of a conclusive diagnosis.

130. The answer is E (all). *(Braunwald, ed 11. pp 657–659.)* Lyme disease was first recognized in 1975 when a clustering of cases of erythema chronicum migrans associated with arthritis occurred around the southern Connecticut town of Lyme. This disease is of particular interest as it is the first arthritis known quite definitely to be triggered by an infectious agent that is associated in many patients with numerous severe chronic complications. In 1983 the organism responsible was identified as a spirochete that can be grown on Kelly's medium. High titers of IgM antibodies to this spirochete develop early in the disease and are virtually diagnostic. A few patients with infectious mononucleosis have developed similar antibodies, although in this case they are probably reactive rather than specific. The disease may not be a new one, as similar cases have probably been described in Europe over the last 50 years and certainly in recent times cases have been described in Europe and Australia. Lyme disease has been found in California, Wisconsin, Connecticut, and New York. Although a lymphocytic meningoradiculitis has been found in Europe to be caused by direct invasion of a spirochete that seems identical to the one that causes Lyme arthritis, many of the complications of this disease may be autoimmune in nature. There are numerous immunological abnormalities in patients with Lyme disease, which is therefore a particularly valuable model for studying the way an environmental agent can disturb immunoregulation. Cardiac conduction abnormalities occur in a small number of patients, but they can be severe, ranging from first degree to complete heart block. The neurological complications consist most commonly of an aseptic meningitis but also encephalitis and cranial nerve disorders. A radiculoneuritis and myelitis have been observed. Tetracycline and penicillin are equally good at blocking the early stages of the disease, but tetracycline treatment appears to minimize the development of chronic complications involving the heart and nervous system.

131. The answer is E (all). *(Braunwald, ed 11. pp 1433–1434.)* Sjögren's syndrome consists of the triad of keratoconjunctivitis sicca, xerostomia, and a connective tissue disorder. The diagnosis is warranted when two of these three features are present. The connective tissue disease most commonly associated with the sicca complex is rheumatoid arthritis, but other diseases such as systemic lupus erythematosus, scleroderma, polymyositis, chronic active hepatitis, Waldenström's macroglobulinemia, pseudolymphoma, and malignant lymphoma also may be a part of this complex. A group of patients afflicted with Sjögren's syndrome has been identified as having only the sicca complex (dry eyes and mouth). In this group, systemic complaints such as fatigue and arthralgias may be present.

132. The answer is D (4). *(Braunwald, ed 11. pp 1286–1287, 1460–1461.)* The peripheral arthritis associated with inflammatory bowel disease is found in approximately 25 percent of cases, more commonly in Crohn's disease and especially when the regional enteritis involves the colon. The arthritis is nondeforming, monoarticular or polyarticular, without definite symmetry, and migratory. The attacks may be acute and most frequently involve the knees and ankles, although any joint may be affected. Serologic tests are negative and synovial fluid findings are typical of an acute arthritis. Attacks usually parallel the disease activity of the colitis. Prognostically, complete resolution without deformities occurs within several weeks. This is in contrast to the ankylosing spondylitis of inflammatory bowel disease, which commonly precedes the colitis and progresses regardless of the course of the underlying gastrointestinal dysfunction.

133–137. The answers are: 133-B, 134-A, 135-E, 136-C, 137-D. *(Braunwald, ed 11, p 1455.)* Examination of the synovial fluid may provide specific diagnostic information in infectious arthritis, gout, pseudogout, and in neoplastic diseases involving joints. Normal joint fluid is clear and colorless, has less than 200 white blood cells/mm³ (most of which are mononuclear), and has a high viscosity. The viscosity, which correlates with the mucin clot, can be evaluated by observing a drop of synovial fluid released from a syringe. A normal viscosity will exhibit a string of fluid several inches long; fluid of diminished viscosity will behave like water.

Traumatic arthritis and osteoarthritis are usually associated with synovial fluid white blood cell counts of less than 2000/mm³. In rheumatoid arthritis, Reiter's syndrome, gout, pseudogout, and other inflammatory forms of arthritis, synovial fluid white blood cell counts usually are in the range of 20,000 to 60,000/mm³; in patients with pyogenic arthritis, white blood cell counts are frequently higher, especially when the infecting organisms are staphylococci or streptococci.

Synovial fluid complement levels may be helpful in distinguishing among some inflammatory forms of arthritis. Normal synovial fluid has a relatively low complement level in relation to the complement level in the blood because the large complement molecules do not easily penetrate the synovial membrane. When inflammation occurs, the synovium becomes more permeable, and complement components can then readily enter the joint space. In diseases such as rheumatoid arthritis, immune complexes are formed in synovial fluid. These complexes lead to complement activation; consequently, complement levels are decreased. Other inflammatory diseases, such as Reiter's syndrome, appear not to be associated with intraarticular complement consumption and are distinguished by having elevated complement levels.

In patients who have gout, synovial fluid examined by polarized light microscopy reveals negatively birefringent needle-shaped urate crystals; in pseudogout, smaller, more rhomboid-shaped crystals that exhibit weakly positive birefringence are seen.

138–142. The answers are: 138-A, 139-C, 140-D, 141-B, 142-B. *(Braunwald, ed 11. pp 1423–1428.)* Drugs used for the suppression of inflammation of rheumatoid arthritis are broadly classified as immunosuppressive drugs, remission-inducing agents, and anti-inflammatory agents. Indomethacin (Indocin), a nonsteroidal anti-inflammatory agent that inhibits prostaglandin synthesis, is a commonly used first-line drug. The most frequent side effects include gastrointestinal distress and headaches.

Gold therapy is effective in most patients with rheumatoid arthritis, especially in those whose disease is of recent onset. Side effects, however, are significant and include a dermatitis that may lead to exfoliative dermatitis if treatment is not discontinued, the nephrotic syndrome, and bone marrow suppression.

Penicillamine is generally used after failure with gold has been demonstrated. Side effects include altered taste sensation, bone marrow suppression, proteinuria, and various autoimmune disorders such as systemic lupus erythematosus and myasthenia gravis.

The most significant side effect of chloroquine is irreversible retinal degeneration, which inhibits the long-term use of this drug. Ophthalmic examinations are required every 6 months of therapy.

143–147. The answers are: 143-C, 144-B, 145-A, 146-A, 147-B. *(Braunwald, ed 11. pp 1436–1437.)* Reiter's syndrome is characterized as a triad of seronegative, oligoarticular, asymmetric arthritis; conjunctivitis; and urethritis; although the arthritis coupled with urethritis or cervicitis may be sufficient for the diagnosis. It is the most common cause of arthritis in young men. The syndrome develops in up to 3 percent of males with nongonococcal urethritis, in 2 to 3 percent of patients with bacillary dysentery, and in 20 percent of persons with the HLA-B27 antigen. While the pathogenesis is unclear, an infectious process of the urogenital tract or gut together with a particular genetic background may trigger the development of Reiter's syndrome.

The disorder usually begins with urethritis followed by conjunctivitis, which is usually minimal, and rheumatologic findings. The arthritis is usually acute, asymmetric, and oligoarticular and involves predominantly the joints of the lower extremities; tenosynovitis, dactylitis, and plantar fasciitis also occur. Painless, superficial oral mucosal and glans penile lesions occur in a third of patients; keratosis blennorrhagica occurs in up to 30 percent of postvenereal Reiter's syndrome patients but does not occur in postdysentery patients; circinate balanitis is a characteristic dermatitis of the glans penis.

The diagnosis of gonococcal arthritis is made if the organism is cultured from a mucosal site, typical pustular or hemorrhagic lesions are distributed primarily on the extremities, and a therapeutic antibiotic trial resolves the fevers and arthritis. The course is typically acute, typically involves joints of the upper extremities, and may be associated with uveitis.

Pulmonary Disease

DIRECTIONS: The questions below contain five suggested responses. Select the **one best** response to each question.

148. A 64-year-old woman is found to have a left-sided pleural effusion on chest x-ray. Analysis of the pleural fluid reveals a ratio of concentration of total protein in pleural fluid to serum of 0.38, a lactic dehydrogenase (LDH) level of 125 IU, and a ratio of LDH concentration in pleural fluid to serum of 0.46. Which of the following disorders is most likely in this patient?

(A) Uremia
(B) Congestive heart failure
(C) Pulmonary embolism
(D) Sarcoidosis
(E) Systemic lupus erythematosus

149. A patient is found to have an unexpectedly high value for diffusing capacity. This finding is consistent with which of the following disorders?

(A) Anemia
(B) Cystic fibrosis
(C) Emphysema
(D) Intrapulmonary hemorrhage
(E) Pulmonary emboli

150. All the following statements concerning the pulmonary effects of radiation therapy are true EXCEPT

(A) symptoms of radiation pneumonitis usually become evident 2 to 3 months after the completion of radiation therapy
(B) frank hemoptysis is an uncommon symptom of radiation pneumonitis
(C) radiation fibrosis usually establishes itself no less than 3 years after completion of radiation therapy
(D) the earliest radiologic change after irradiation of the thorax is a radiolucency of the irradiated area
(E) a second course of radiation therapy to the lung is more likely to precipitate acute radiation pneumonitis than the first

151. Goodpasture's syndrome, a rare
cause of pulmonary disease, is characterized by which of the following statements?

(A) It is a contraindication to renal
transplantation
(B) Decreased levels of complement
components are typical
(C) The level of antibody to basement
membrane correlates with the severity of the disease
(D) It is associated with a hypochromic, microcytic anemia that is out
of proportion to the degree of
hemoptysis
(E) The nephrotic syndrome is
common

DIRECTIONS: Each question below contains four suggested responses of which **one or more** is correct. Select

A	if	**1, 2, and 3**	are correct
B	if	**1 and 3**	are correct
C	if	**2 and 4**	are correct
D	if	**4**	is correct
E	if	**1, 2, 3, and 4**	are correct

152. A 28-year-old man enters the hospital with cough and fever. His admission x-ray is shown below. Acid-fast organisms, subsequently identified as *Mycobacterium tuberculosis,* are identified on a smear. Correct statements regarding the pathophysiology of this patient's infection include which of the following?

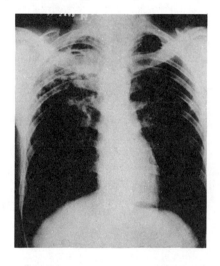

(1) The initial exposure probably occurred at a time remote from the current symptoms
(2) The location of the current process probably resulted from inspiration of aerosolized droplets into the upper lobe
(3) Necrosis of the pulmonary lesion with cavity formation is a common complication of his condition
(4) Risk of infection to hospital staff will be reduced if the patient is kept on an open, well-ventilated ward

153. The changes in lung function seen with aging include

(1) an increase in ventilation-perfusion mismatch
(2) a decrease in vital capacity
(3) a decrease in forced expiratory volume
(4) a decrease in functional residual capacity

154. Respiratory alkalosis is associated with which of the following?

(1) An increase in the urinary excretion of phosphate
(2) A renal compensation that is faster than the renal response to acute hypercapnia
(3) Lactic acid generation to levels greater than 5 mEq/L
(4) Cirrhosis of the liver

155. Correct statements concerning oxygen toxicity include which of the following?

(1) Breathing 100% oxygen may result in a large right-to-left shunt
(2) Changes in pulmonary function tests are not seen when lungs are exposed to less than 0.5 atmospheres
(3) Pulmonary fibrosis may occur after 1 week of exposure to an FI_{O_2} of 1.0
(4) The risk of retrolental fibroplasia is not directly related to the inspired FI_{O_2}

156. True statements concerning theophylline include that

(1) at therapeutic concentrations, inhibition of phosphodiesterase activity is insignificant
(2) cimetidine causes a marked decrease in theophylline clearance
(3) it augments the ventilatory response to hypoxia
(4) it appears in breast milk in significant concentrations

157. A 36-year-old woman with sarcoidosis has been managed conservatively for 1 year. During this period, despite radiographic evidence of extensive lung involvement, she has not had significant respiratory symptoms. She now complains of some exertional dyspnea associated with a cough and her physician reevaluates her case. Her chest x-ray shows little change. Pulmonary function tests are reported to show restrictive lung disease. Which of the following abnormalities would support the diagnosis of restrictive lung disease?

(1) A decrease in flow rates at midvital capacity compared with predicted values
(2) An increase in FEV_1/FVC ratio
(3) An increase in functional residual capacity
(4) An increase in the alveolar-arterial oxygen tension difference

158. Severe kyphoscoliosis is associated with which of the following pulmonary abnormalities?

(1) Increased ventilation-perfusion mismatch
(2) Reduced diffusing capacity
(3) Decreased functional residual capacity
(4) Reduced dynamic lung compliance

159. True statements concerning the pulmonary involvement in Wegener's granulomatosis include that

(1) hilar adenopathy is commonly the initial chest x-ray abnormality
(2) lung volumes remain unchanged until late in the illness
(3) calcification of granulomata is a frequent finding
(4) multiple, bilateral nodal infiltrates are typical

160. Lung abscesses are characterized by which of the following statements?

(1) An associated empyema indicates the presence of a bronchopleural fistula
(2) They rarely occur in an edentulous person
(3) Surgical resection reduces the length of antibiotic therapy
(4) Cavities appear an average of 12 days after aspiration

161. True statements concerning complications of tracheostomies include which of the following?

(1) Airway colonization with *Pseudomonas* or gram-negative enteric organisms occurs in the majority of patients
(2) Nosocomial pneumonia occurs more frequently in patients with prolonged endotracheal intubation than in those with tracheostomies
(3) Symptoms of tracheal stenosis may develop years after extubation
(4) Pneumothorax will not occur because the tracheal incision is far from the pleura

162. The physiologic dynamics of a spontaneous pneumothorax are characterized by which of the following statements?

(1) Lung collapse occurs because intrabronchial pressures are greater than intrapleural pressures
(2) Hypoxemia is secondary to ventilation-perfusion mismatch
(3) A positive intrapleural pressure of 15 cmH_2O may reduce cardiac output
(4) Diffusing capacity is not reduced

DIRECTIONS: Each group of questions below consists of lettered headings followed by a set of numbered items. For each numbered item select the **one** lettered heading with which it is **most** closely associated. Each lettered heading may be used **once, more than once, or not at all.**

Questions 163–167

For each clinical picture below, select the arterial blood gas and pH values with which it is most likely to be associated.

	pH	P_{O_2}	P_{CO_2}
(A)	7.54	75	28
(B)	7.15	78	92
(C)	7.06	36	95
(D)	7.30	58	44
(E)	7.39	48	54

163. A 30-year-old obese female bus driver develops sudden pleuritic left-sided chest pain and dyspnea

164. A 60-year-old heavy smoker has severe chronic bronchitis and peripheral edema and cyanosis

165. A 22-year-old drug-addicted man is brought to the emergency room by friends who were unable to awaken him

166. A 62-year-old man who has chronic bronchitis and chest pain is given oxygen via mask in the ambulance en route to the hospital and becomes lethargic in the emergency room

167. A 20-year-old man brought to the emergency room is still wheezing 18 hours later despite vigorous therapy for episodic asthma

Questions 168–172

For each set of findings below, select the disease with which it is most likely to be associated.

(A) Asthma
(B) Rheumatoid arthritis
(C) α_1-Antitrypsin deficiency
(D) Cystic fibrosis
(E) Bronchiectasis

168. High levels of lactic dehydrogenase in pleural effusions

169. Decreased synthesis of prostaglandins

170. Presence of the mucoid strain of *Pseudomonas aeruginosa*

171. Development of severe liver disease that is usually associated with, but may be independent of, lung disease

172. Progressive dyspnea, but very little coughing

DIRECTIONS: The group of questions below consists of four lettered headings followed by a set of numbered items. For each numbered item select

A	if the item is associated with	(A) **only**
B	if the item is associated with	(B) **only**
C	if the item is associated with	**both** (A) and (B)
D	if the item is associated with	**neither** (A) nor (B)

Each lettered heading may be used **once, more than once, or not at all.**

Questions 173–177

    (A) Rheumatoid arthritis
    (B) Scleroderma
    (C) Both
    (D) Neither

173. Acute pneumonia
174. Diffuse interstitial fibrosis
175. Pleural effusion
176. Pulmonary nodules
177. Primary pulmonary vasculopathy

Pulmonary Disease

Answers

148. The answer is B. *(Fishman, ed 2. p 2134.)* Classifying a pleural effusion as either a transudate or an exudate is useful in identifying the underlying disorder. Pleural fluid is exudative if it has any one of the following three properties: a ratio of concentration of total protein in pleural fluid to serum greater than 0.5, an absolute value of LDH greater than 200 IU, or a ratio of LDH concentration in pleural fluid to serum greater than 0.6. Causes of exudative effusions include malignancy, pulmonary embolism, parapneumonia, tuberculosis, abdominal disease, collagen vascular diseases, uremia, Dressler's syndrome, and chylothorax, and exudative effusions may also be drug-induced. If none of the aforementioned properties are met, the effusion is a transudate. Differential diagnosis includes congestive heart failure, nephrotic syndrome, cirrhosis, Meigs's syndrome, and hydronephrosis. It is important to note that congestive heart failure, pneumonia, malignancy, and pulmonary embolic disease account for more than 90 percent of all pleural effusions.

149. The answer is D. *(Fishman, ed 2. p 2497.)* The diffusing capacity provides an estimate of the rate at which carbon monoxide moves by diffusion from alveolar gas to combine with hemoglobin in the red blood cells. It is interpreted as an index of the surface area engaged in alveolar-capillary diffusion. Measurement of diffusing capacity of the lung (DL_{CO}) is done by having the person inspire a low concentration of carbon monoxide. The rate of uptake of the gas by the blood is calculated from the difference between the inspired and expired concentrations. The test can be performed during a single 10-second breath-holding or during a minute of steady-state breathing. The diffusing capacity is defined as the amount of carbon monoxide transferred per minute per millimeter of mercury of driving pressure. Normal values hover about 20 (ml/min)/mm Hg at rest and 60 (ml/min)/mm Hg on exercise. Primary parenchymal disorders and removal of lung tissue decrease the diffusing surface area and cause the DL_{CO} to be low. Conversely, polycythemia and intrapulmonary hemorrhage tend to increase the value for diffusing capacity.

150. The answer is C. *(Gross, Ann Intern Med 86:81–92, 1977.)* Radiation administered to the thorax in the treatment of patients with breast cancer, lung cancer, Hodgkin's disease, or lymphoma may result in adverse effects on lung and pleura. The incidence and severity of damage are related to two major factors: the greater the volume of lung irradiated, the greater the likelihood of clinical disturbance; and the amount of damage produced is more a function of the rate at which the total dose is delivered than of the total dose, as increasing fractionation allows repair of sublethal damage. The clinical syndrome is divided into two phases: radiation pneumonitis, which occurs 2 to 6 months after radiation therapy, and radiation fibrosis, which follows it and is usually established by 12 months. Symptoms of radiation pneumonitis begin insidiously and usually consist of a harsh cough and dyspnea; frank hemoptysis is uncommon. Nearly all patients with radiation pneumonitis will develop radiation fibrosis and in most cases this will be asymptomatic. However, in severe cases, dyspnea, orthopnea, cyanosis, and finger clubbing may occur. Concomitant chemotherapy, repeat courses of radiation, and steroid withdrawal all may potentiate the damaging effects of radiation. Interestingly, while dactinomycin, cyclophosphamide, and vincristine enhance the lethality of thoracic irradiation, hydroxyurea and bleomycin do not.

151. The answer is D. *(Braunwald, ed 11. pp 1185–1186.)* Goodpasture's syndrome is a disease characterized by pulmonary hemorrhages, nephritis, and anti-basement-membrane antibody. It usually occurs in young adult males. Hemoptysis is the most common pulmonary manifestation and it tends to be recurrent, ranging from mild to life-threatening. Commonly, the renal disease is progressive and may lead to oliguric renal failure in just a few weeks. Systemic symptoms at the time of presentation are unremarkable. Laboratory studies reveal circulating antibody to basement-membrane antigens in over 90 percent of patients; complement levels are normal. Immunofluorescence of renal and lung biopsies reveals linear deposits of antibody along the basement membranes. The course of the disease is highly variable and treatment involves steroids, cytotoxic drugs, and plasmapheresis. Goodpasture's syndrome is not a contraindication to renal transplantation providing anti-basement-membrane antibodies reach undetectable levels.

152. The answer is B (1, 3). *(Braunwald, ed 11. pp 625–627.)* The patient described in the question has postprimary tuberculosis. The causative organism is initially inhaled by droplet aerosol into the lower lobes where ventilation is high. A primary, usually asymptomatic, infection ensues. Organisms are spread subsequently by hematogenous dissemination to other foci and grow best in those areas with a high oxygen tension, such as the upper lobe. Necrosis is part of the characteristic tissue reaction to infection. Symptomatic disease may then occur at these distant locations later in life. As the organism spreads by droplet aerosol, isolation of the patient becomes mandatory, preferably in a room with ultraviolet radiation.

153. The answer is A (1, 2, 3). *(Braunwald, ed 11. p 1055.)* It has been shown that the P_{O_2} falls in an almost linear fashion with age predominantly because of an increasing ventilation-perfusion mismatch. Other changes that occur include an increase in the functional residual capacity, residual volume, and closing volume and a decrease in the vital capacity and forced expiratory volume.

154. The answer is C (2, 4). *(Arieff, pp 393–400.)* Respiratory alkalosis is an acid-base disturbance characterized by hypocapnia and a compensatory bicarbonate diuresis and acid retention. Causes include congestive heart failure, pneumonia, pulmonary embolism, asthma, progesterone, salicylates, cirrhosis, fever, and subarachnoid hemorrhage. It is typically accompanied by hypophosphatemia caused by cellular shift, a reduction in the excretion of phosphate, hypokalemia, and generation of lactic acid. The rise in blood lactate, however, is small and concentrations above 5 mEq/L should initiate a search for other causes.

155. The answer is E (all). *(Miller, ed 2. pp 1151, 1157.)* Pulmonary oxygen toxicity is related to both the tension of administered oxygen and the duration of exposure. While human trials are not possible, indirect analyses have lead to several conclusions: Oxygen toxicity does not occur in patients exposed to less than 0.5 atmospheres, and an $F_{I_{O_2}}$ of 1.0 should not be given for greater than 12 hours duration. Furthermore, an $F_{I_{O_2}}$ of 1.0 may actually decrease arterial O_2 content by causing absorption atelectasis in those regions of the lung with low V/Q ratios. With time, exposure to a high $F_{I_{O_2}}$ causes a tracheobronchitis that progresses within a few days to pulmonary interstitial edema and finally to pulmonary fibrosis. Retrolental fibroplasia is a complication seen in infants of less than 1.0 kg birth weight and 28 weeks gestation and is characterized by a proliferation of retinal vasculature in response to hyperoxia. The risk is significant whenever the $F_{I_{O_2}}$ causes a Pa_{O_2} of greater than 80 mm Hg; this complication, then, is directly related to the Pa_{O_2} and not the inspired $F_{I_{O_2}}$.

156. The answer is A (1, 2, 3). *(Bukowskyj, Ann Intern Med 101:63–73, 1984.)* Theophylline, a methylxanthine, is a frequently used drug in airway obstruction. One of its effects is to inhibit phosphodiesterase activity; however, at therapeutic concentrations, this inhibition is minimal and inadequate to explain the bronchodilation seen. More plausible in explaining theophylline's therapeutic effects is its ability to antagonize adenosine activity. Adenosine, a known bronchoconstrictor, is structurally similar to theophylline. The competitive inhibition of adenosine receptors occurs in a dose-dependent fashion and in theophylline's therapeutic range. Other effects of theophylline include improvement of diaphragmatic contractility and augmentation of the ventilatory response to hypoxia. Theophylline metabolism is altered by many drugs. Cimetidine, erythromycin, and birth control pills all reduce its clearance, while phenobarbital and dilantin increase its clearance. Theophylline readily crosses the placenta but only 1 percent of the maternal dose appears in breast milk. Teratogenicity has not been described.

157. The answer is C (2, 4). *(Braunwald, ed 11. pp 1053–1055, 1447.)* Sarcoidosis runs an unpredictable course. The lesions may spontaneously resolve or begin to organize and promote scarring that can disrupt the alveoli and produce restrictive lung disease. Evidence of such a course would be an indication for treatment with corticosteroids. Reliable information can be gained from pulmonary function tests. Restrictive lung disease is characterized by a decrease in total lung capacity. The associated decrease in the alveolar surface area, together with ventilation-perfusion inequality, diminishes the diffusing capacity and increases alveolar-arterial oxygen differences. The FEV_1 is supernormal early in the disease and well maintained even in advanced disease; the forced vital capacity falls, however. Thus, the FEV_1/FVC ratio tends to rise. Despite the fall in lung volume, flow rates over the middle portion of the FEV curve continue within the normal range. The functional residual capacity and the residual volume are increased in diseases, such as chronic bronchitis, that are characterized by increased airway resistance.

158. The answer is E (all). *(Fishman, ed 2. pp 2301, 2509.)* Patients with severe kyphoscoliosis may demonstrate a respiratory insufficiency so severe as to lead to cor pulmonale and respiratory failure. Hypoxemia is attributed to both ventilation-perfusion mismatch and hypoventilation. Diffusing capacity is often severely reduced and parallels the decrease in vital capacity and total lung capacity. Pectus excavatum and spondylitis may also cause dyspnea, but respiratory failure does not occur.

159. The answer is D (4). *(Fauci, Ann Intern Med 98:76–85, 1983.)* Wegener's granulomatosis is characterized by glomerulonephritis together with a granulomatous vasculitis of the upper and lower respiratory tracts. Patients typically present with an upper airway illness related to persistent rhinorrhea and bilateral pulmonary infiltrates. Rarely is there functional renal impairment on presentation. Lung biopsy reveals the presence of granulomata and vasculitis, although, rarely, either may exist alone. The characteristic lung findings are multiple, bilateral nodal infiltrates that tend to cavitate. Twenty percent of patients have pleural effusions. Pulmonary calcifications are rare and hilar adenopathy is not a feature. On pulmonary function testing, airflow obstruction, reduced lung volumes, and an abnormal diffusing capacity are common findings. Without therapy, mortality is 90 percent in 2 years. Treatment with prednisone and cyclophosphamide or azathioprine achieves complete remission in over 90 percent of patients.

160. The answer is C (2, 4). *(Mandell, ed 2. pp 407–411.)* Lung abscess is characterized by destruction of lung parenchyma secondary to a suppurative inflammatory process resulting in cavitary lesions. Frequent predisposing factors include aspiration, periodontal disease, bronchiectasis, bacteremia, and intraabdominal infection. Anaerobic abscesses typically have an indolent course while those caused by *Staphylococcus aureus, Streptococcus pyogenes,* or *Klebsiella* have a more sudden presentation. Lung abscesses secondary to another process such as bacterial endocarditis or subphrenic infection may be dominated by the clinical presentation of the underlying pathology. Approximately one-third of lung abscesses are complicated by empyema, which may occur in the absence of a detectable fistula. Treatment involves 2 to 4 months of antimicrobial therapy for complete resolution; surgical resection is contraindicated unless a malignant process is present.

161.   The answer is B (1, 3). *(Heffner, Chest 90:269–273, 430–435, 1986.)* Tracheostomy is one of the more frequent surgical procedures; indications include upper airway obstruction, long-term mechanical ventilation, and weaning from mechanical ventilation. While mortality is less than 2 percent, a number of complications are recognized. Because pleural extension into the neck may occur, especially in patients with emphysema, pneumothorax is not uncommon and develops in up to 5 percent of patients. Nosocomial pneumonias are more common and more serious in patients with tracheostomies than in those with prolonged endotracheal intubation and commonly involve *Pseudomonas* and gram-negative enteric organisms. Tracheal stenoses result from excessive cuff pressures and form as the tracheal injury heals. They manifest as dyspnea on exertion, cough, difficulty in clearing secretions, and stridor and may present several months to several years after extubation. Various forms of bleeding and tracheoesophageal fistulas are other noted complications.

162.   The answer is A (1, 2, 3). *(Braunwald, ed 11. pp 1126–1127.)* Intrabronchial pressure within the lungs remains greater than intrapleural pressure throughout the respiratory cycle as a consequence of elastic recoil of the lung. When a pulmonary cyst ruptures, air moves into the pleural cavity causing a loss of intrapleural pressure and collapse of the lung. The process stops when the leak seals or when the two pressures equalize. Hypoxemia, secondary to continued perfusion of nonventilated areas, is usually transient as perfusion of the collapsed lung decreases with time. Lung volumes, compliance, and diffusion capacity are all reduced. A tension pneumothorax is produced when, as a result of a ball-valve effect, air progressively enters the pleural space during expiration when intrabronchial pressures increase. Because venous blood return is inhibited, cardiac output drops.

163–167.   The answers are: 163-A, 164-E, 165-C, 166-B, 167-D. *(Braunwald, ed 11. pp 1053–1055. Guenter, ed 2. pp 119, 482, 722, 724.)* The blood gas values associated with pulmonary embolism may vary tremendously. It is important to note that hypoxemia need not be present, as illustrated in the laboratory values accompanying the question.

   In severe chronic lung disease, the presence of hypercapnia leads to a compensatory increase in serum bicarbonate. Thus, significant hypercapnia may be present with an arterial pH close to normal.

   Acute respiratory acidosis may occur secondary to respiratory depression after drug overdose. Hypoventilation is associated with hypoxia, hypercapnia, and severe, uncompensated acidosis.

   In the presence of long-standing lung disease, respiration may become regulated by hypoxia rather than by altered carbon dioxide tension and arterial pH, as in normal people. Thus, the unmonitored administration of oxygen may lead to respiratory suppression, as in the patient described in the question.

In asthmatic episodes, significant hypoxia is not uncommon. After 18 hours, an affected patient's strength may be waning so that eucapnia or hypercapnia may be present rather than the hypocapnia characteristic of respiratory alkalosis; this normalization of P_{CO_2} signals the onset of respiratory failure.

168–172. The answers are: 168-B, 169-A, 170-D, 171-C, 172-C. *(Braunwald, ed 11. pp 1060–1063, 1082–1086, 1088, 1125.)* Pleural effusions are not unusual in patients with rheumatoid arthritis. A history of pleurodynia that would suggest an antecedent inflammatory pleuritis is not always obtained, but characteristically the pleural fluid, which is sterile, will contain a high level of lactic dehydrogenase and a low glucose concentration. Other pulmonary phenomena associated with rheumatoid arthritis include diffuse interstitial fibrosis and the occurrence of individual or clustered nodules in the lung parenchyma.

Asthma is frequently associated with bronchiolitis and immediate hypersensitivity reactions, but it should be kept in mind that exercise and intolerance to certain anti-inflammatory agents also are common triggering mechanisms for reversible airway obstruction. Fifteen percent of patients with asthma will experience bronchospasm shortly after the ingestion of aspirin or indomethacin, but not sodium salicylate. Other compounds that can produce the same effect, such as tartrazine yellow, the food coloring agent found in many drugs and as a coloring additive in over 200 food products, may be extremely difficult to avoid. Recent evidence suggests that in such patients these compounds are able to block cyclooxygenase activity needed to facilitate the reduction of arachidonic acid to prostaglandins. In the absence of this pathway, increased amounts of slow-reacting substance of anaphylaxis are produced.

The fatality rate for patients with cystic fibrosis is lower today than in previous years; currently, the average life span of patients afflicted with this disease is 19 years. Chronic lung infections, however, are almost universal. The most common and difficult to treat of such infections is caused by the mucoid strain of *Pseudomonas aeruginosa*. It is doubtful whether any form of antibiotic combination is effective in such patients. Distressing and chronic coughing is one of the major problems of patients with cystic fibrosis. Liver disease, particularly biliary cirrhosis, may develop in patients afflicted with *Pseudomonas aeruginosa* infections and about 3 percent of these patients present with portal hypertension.

The incidence of liver disease associated with a deficiency of α_1-antitrypsin is much higher than with *Pseudomonas aeruginosa* infections. Indeed, it is estimated that 15 percent of all chronic liver disease is associated with this deficiency. Panacinar emphysema with very little coughing is the predominant feature of lung involvement.

173–177. The answers are: 173-D, 174-C, 175-A, 176-A, 177-B. *(Fishman, ed 2. p 646.)* Rheumatoid arthritis is a chronic inflammatory disease characterized by a symmetric polyarthritis affecting the small joints of the hands and feet as well as the large peripheral joints. Systemic features include fever, malaise, weight loss, and easy fatigability. Laboratory abnormalities include a normocytic, hypochromic anemia, diffuse hypergammaglobulinemia, hypoalbuminemia, and an elevated erythrocyte sedimentation rate. The pulmonary manifestations recognized to be part of the syndrome of rheumatoid arthritis are pleurisy with or without effusion, intrapulmonary rheumatoid nodules, rheumatoid pneumoconiosis, diffuse interstitial fibrosis, and brochiolitis; ventilatory insufficiency is rare.

Scleroderma is a systemic, often progressive disorder of connective tissue. Presenting manifestations usually include Raynaud's phenomenon, thickening of the skin of the fingers, or musculoskeletal symptoms. The visceral organs affected include the gastrointestinal tract, kidneys, heart, and lungs. Pulmonary manifestations are pleural thickening, diffuse interstitial fibrosis, primary pulmonary vasculopathy, and ventilatory insufficiency. The diffusing capacity is low and the lung volumes are decreased; respiratory failure is a rare but important consequence of pulmonary disease in scleroderma.

Cardiology

DIRECTIONS: Each question below contains five suggested responses. Select the **one best** response to each question.

178. A 24-year-old man approaches his doctor to discuss the assessment of his physical training regimen. He is training to be a marathon runner and he wishes to know how his cardiovascular system should respond to his strenuous exercise. His physician could document all EXCEPT which of the following statements?

(A) Successful physical training will dramatically lower heart rate at rest

(B) Maximal increase in cardiac performance can be achieved by exercising large muscle groups three to five times per week such that 60 percent of the maximum heart rate is obtained and maintained for at least 15 minutes

(C) The percentage of maximal oxygen uptake (V_{o2max}) is the best overall measurement of the efficiency of training

(D) With training, peripheral muscles (e.g., calf muscles) will demand less oxygen per unit of work performed

(E) If only the legs are involved in vigorous training exercises only the legs will benefit from the circulatory adaptive changes that enhance muscle performance

179. A 25-year-old woman is seen by her physician because of progressive dyspnea, fatigue, and syncope on exertion. She has no history of rheumatic fever or heart murmur. The patient was in excellent health until 6 months ago when her symptoms developed; they have since become progressively worse. Physical examination reveals a well-developed, well-nourished, acyanotic woman who experiences mild respiratory distress at rest. The jugular pulse reveals large α waves. There is a prominent right ventricular heave. A palpable pulmonic closure is present and a grade III/VI systolic ejection murmur is heard at the left second intercostal space. A grade I/VI blowing, holosystolic murmur is also noted at the lower left sternal border. The pulmonic closure is loud but splits normally with inspiration. The electrocardiogram reveals right ventricular hypertrophy. A chest x-ray shows dilation of the main pulmonary arteries with decreased vascularity in the outer one-third of the lung fields. The most likely diagnosis is which of the following?

(A) Atrial septal defect

(B) Ventricular septal defect

(C) Congenital pulmonic stenosis

(D) Tetralogy of Fallot

(E) Primary pulmonary hypertension

180. All the following statements concerning intracardiac thrombi are true EXCEPT

(A) left ventricular thrombi are more common after anterior than after inferior infarction
(B) thrombi usually develop within the first week after infarction
(C) left ventricular thrombi in patients with idiopathic dilated cardiomyopathy frequently embolize
(D) left atrial enlargement is a predisposing factor to formation of left atrial thrombi
(E) intraaneurysmal left ventricular thrombi have a high frequency of embolization

---

181. The rhythm strip displayed below reveals

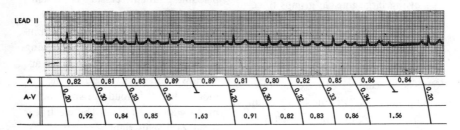

LEAD II										
A	0.82	0.81	0.83	0.89	0.89	0.81	0.80	0.82	0.85	0.86	0.84
A-V	0.28	0.30	0.33	0.35		0.28	0.30	0.32	0.33	0.34	0.28
V	0.92	0.84	0.85	1.63		0.91	0.82	0.83	0.86	1.56

(A) atrial premature contractions
(B) junctional premature contractions
(C) AV dissociation
(D) type I AV block
(E) type II AV block

182. A 43-year-old woman with a 1-year history of episodic leg edema and dyspnea is noted to have clubbing of the fingers. Her ECG is shown below. The correct diagnosis is

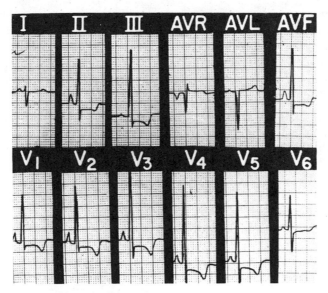

(A) inferior wall myocardial infarction
(B) right bundle branch block
(C) anterior wall myocardial infarction
(D) Wolff-Parkinson-White syndrome
(E) cor pulmonale

183. All the following statements concerning the rhythm strip displayed below are true EXCEPT

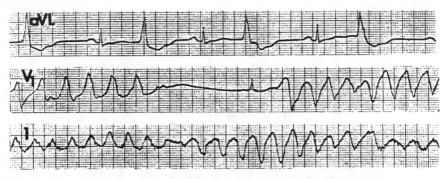

(A) it is usually initiated by a premature ventricular contraction in the presence of a long Q-T interval
(B) it most frequently results from drug administration
(C) once the arrhythmia is terminated by ventricular pacing, prophylaxis with quinidine is appropriate therapy
(D) it is associated with bradycardia, particularly when caused by AV block
(E) it may degenerate to ventricular fibrillation

184. For a tachycardia with a widened QRS complex; which of the following electrocardiographic findings favors a ventricular versus a supraventricular origin?

(A) Right bundle branch block–shaped QRS complexes at a frequency above 170/min
(B) AV dissociation during tachycardia
(C) Alternation in the R-R interval during tachycardia
(D) Right axis deviation in the frontal plane
(E) Triphasic right bundle branch block–shaped QRS complexes in lead V_1

185. The electrocardiogram displayed below reveals which of the following patterns?

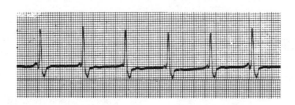

(A) Normal sinus rhythm
(B) Junctional or nodal rhythm
(C) Idioventricular rhythm
(D) Complete heart block
(E) Atrioventricular dissociation

186. Which of the following statements correctly describes the most common primary cardiac tumor?

(A) The majority are located in the left ventricle
(B) It occurs more commonly in men than in women
(C) Clinical presentation usually mimics mitral valve disease
(D) It is histologically malignant
(E) Peak incidence occurs in the second decade of life

187. A 45-year-old white man is recovering from his first anterior myocardial infarction. As part of a program to
control this patient's ischemic heart
disease, his doctor discusses with the
patient certain risk factors and how to
avoid them. The physician would be
justified in emphasizing all the following points EXCEPT that

(A) regular exercise can increase high
     density lipoproteins, which are
     known to have a protective effect
     in ischemic heart disease
(B) scientific evidence conclusively
     demonstrates that stopping ciga-
     rette smoking decreases the risk of
     further complications of ischemic
     heart disease
(C) men with normal diastolic blood
     pressures (less than 83 mm Hg)
     but elevated systolic blood pres-
     sure (greater than 158 mm Hg)
     have in excess of a twofold in-
     creased risk of developing severe
     cardiovascular disease compared
     with persons with a normal sys-
     tolic blood pressure
(D) the reduction to normal of diastolic
     blood pressures that lie between 95
     and 105 mm Hg has been clearly
     shown to reduce the risk of cardio-
     vascular morbidity
(E) a family history of xanthomata is
     associated with an increased risk
     of ischemic heart disease

188. Mitral valve prolapse, the most
common abnormality of human heart
valves, is characterized by all the following statements EXCEPT

(A) migration of the systolic click
     and systolic murmur toward the
     first heart sound occurs during
     squatting
(B) echocardiography demonstrates
     posterior displacement of one or
     both mitral valve leaflets
(C) propranolol has been found to be
     helpful in those patients with pal-
     pitations and chest pain
(D) the syndrome appears to be inher-
     ited as an autosomal dominant
     condition with variable penetrance
(E) progression of the valvular defect
     to severe mitral regurgitation that
     necessitates surgical repair may
     occur

189. All the following statements concerning calcium channel blockers are true EXCEPT that

(A) verapamil and diltiazem slow AV conduction

(B) calcium gluconate is recommended for reversing the hypotension of verapamil toxicity

(C) nifedipine has a greater peripheral vasodilator effect than does diltiazem

(D) they are ineffective at therapeutic dosages for decreasing venous capacitance

(E) verapamil is effective in converting atrial fibrillation to normal sinus rhythm

190. A 61-year-old man with mild hypertension but no symptoms is found to have a pulsating mass in the midepigastrium. Continuous ultrasound B scanning confirms the diagnosis of an aneurysm of the abdominal aorta. All the following statements about this disease are true EXCEPT that

(A) there is a 15 to 20 percent chance that the aneurysm will rupture if the diameter is less than 6 cm

(B) the mortality associated with surgery for a ruptured abdominal aortic aneurysm is 50 percent

(C) in the absence of other cardiovascular disease, surgery for small aneurysms (4 to 6 cm in diameter) is not indicated

(D) ultrasound examination will disclose the diameter of the aneurysm

(E) prognosis is most closely linked to the presence of other arteriosclerotic cardiovascular disease

191. The electrocardiogram displayed below is most compatible with which of the following diagnoses?

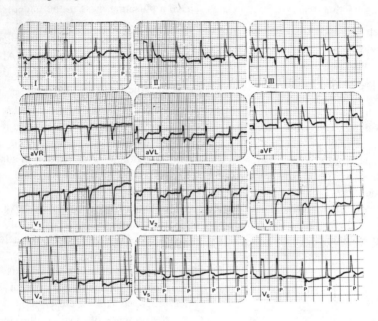

(A) Acute pericarditis with nodal tachycardia
(B) Acute anterior wall myocardial infarction with nodal tachycardia
(C) Acute inferior wall myocardial infarction with nodal tachycardia
(D) Acute inferior wall myocardial infarction with complete heart block
(E) Acute anterolateral myocardial infarction with nodal tachycardia

192. The rhythm strip displayed below demonstrates

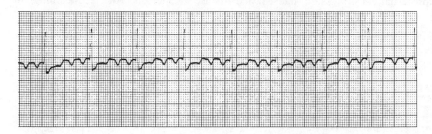

(A) normal sinus rhythm
(B) junctional rhythm
(C) atrial flutter with 4:1 atrioventricular block
(D) paroxysmal atrial tachycardia with 2:1 atrioventricular block
(E) complete heart block with 2:1 atrioventricular block

193. All the following statements concerning the cardiac involvement in malignant carcinoid are true EXCEPT

(A) high cardiac output may occur
(B) a tendency toward pulmonic regurgitation is present
(C) the clinical syndrome is commonly that of tricuspid regurgitation
(D) serotonin antagonists do not affect progression of cardiac lesions
(E) valvular lesions occur only in the presence of hepatic metastases

194. All the following statements about rheumatic fever are true EXCEPT that

(A) the vast majority of patients with carditis do not have symptoms referable to the heart
(B) approximately 75 percent of attacks of acute rheumatic fever subside within 6 weeks
(C) a diagnosis of rheumatic fever without serologic evidence of a recent streptococcal infection is unwarranted
(D) there are no data from controlled clinical trials to suggest that corticosteroids are useful in the treatment of rheumatic carditis
(E) the best antibiotic regimen to prevent recurrence of group A streptococcal infection is the administration of benzathine penicillin, 1.2 million units monthly

195. A 54-year-old man is admitted to the coronary care unit for symptoms of retrosternal chest pressure, nausea, and intense diaphoresis. An electrocardiogram on admission reveals ST-segment elevation in leads V_1 to V_4. An electrocardiogram obtained the following day is shown below. Which of the following steps should next be taken in the management of this patient?

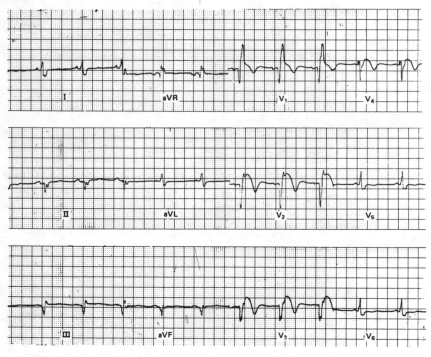

(A) Administration of heparin
(B) Administration of digitalis
(C) Administration of atropine
(D) Temporary transvenous pacing
(E) Observation alone

196. Endocarditis is commonly associated with all the following congenital cardiac lesions EXCEPT

(A) ventricular septal defect
(B) pulmonic stenosis
(C) atrial septal defect
(D) tetralogy of Fallot
(E) patent ductus arteriosus

197. An 82-year-old woman is admitted to the coronary care unit because of episodes of syncope. The patient suddenly becomes unresponsive, and the rhythm strip displayed below is obtained. Pulse and blood pressure are unobtainable. The most appropriate immediate therapy would be to administer

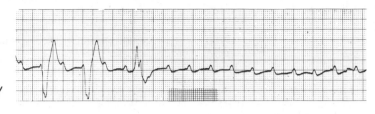

(A) isoproterenol by infusion
(B) norepinephrine by infusion
(C) intravenous lidocaine, 50 mg bolus
(D) intravenous atropine, 1 mg
(E) intracardiac epinephrine

198. A 50-year-old man with a long history of heavy cigarette smoking is admitted to a coronary care unit for an acute inferior wall myocardial infarction. Blood pressure on admission is 140/90 mm Hg, pulse rate 80/minute, and respiratory rate 16/minute. Cardiac examination reveals a loud S_4 gallop only. The patient is given intravenous furosemide, 40 mg, and has a profound diuresis. Twelve hours later, his blood pressure is 80/60 mm Hg and pulse rate 88/minute, and he complains of retrosternal chest pain. A Swan-Ganz pulmonary artery catheter is passed and the patient's pulmonary capillary wedge pressure is 4 mm Hg. The most appropriate immediate therapy would be

(A) infusion of normal saline
(B) infusion of norepinephrine
(C) infusion of dopamine
(D) intravenous furosemide, 40 mg
(E) intravenous nitroglycerin

199. A 45-year-old man is admitted to the hospital for an acute anteroseptal myocardial infarction. Physical examination reveals a blood pressure of 150/100 mm Hg and pulse of 100/minute. The lung fields are clear and cardiac examination reveals only an S_4 gallop. Two days following admission, the patient develops severe shortness of breath. Blood pressure is 100/70 mm Hg, pulse 120/minute, and respiratory rate 32/minute. There are apical rales bilaterally. A grade III/VI systolic murmur is present at the lower left sternal border and both S_3 and S_4 gallops are present. The P_{O_2} is 70 mm Hg. The most likely diagnosis is

(A) pericardial effusion with tamponade
(B) papillary muscle dysfunction
(C) ruptured papillary muscle
(D) rupture of the interventricular septum
(E) acute pulmonary embolus

200. Paradoxical splitting of the second heart sound may occur in association with each of the following cardiovascular disorders EXCEPT

(A) aortic stenosis
(B) right bundle branch block
(C) left bundle branch block
(D) left ventricular ischemia
(E) hypertension

201. On the fifth day of hospitalization for his first myocardial infarction, a 56-year-old man develops mitral regurgitation and left-sided heart failure. Despite treatment with inotropic agents and diuretics over the next 2 weeks, the failure steadily worsens. Although the patient may need surgery, his physicians are anxious to control him medically for at least another 2 weeks. In view of evidence that left ventricular afterload is contributing to this man's heart failure, it has been decided to administer a vasodilator, of which the most suitable in this case would be

(A) nitroglycerine
(B) isosorbide dinitrate
(C) phentolamine
(D) hydralazine
(E) trimethaphan

202. All the following statements regarding coarctation of the aorta are true EXCEPT that

(A) affected patients may complain of leg pain or fatigue
(B) it rarely produces symptoms of congestive heart failure in infancy
(C) it has a higher risk than normal of occurring in patients with Turner's syndrome
(D) it is commonly associated with aortic stenosis due to a bicuspid valve
(E) the lesion usually appears just distal to the left subclavian artery

203. A number of long-term prospective studies of the consequences of different degrees of hypertension and the effects of treatment of this disease have led to firm recommendations regarding medical intervention. Based on the evidence obtained from such studies, all the following statements are accurate EXCEPT that

(A) patients with diastolic blood pressure higher than 105 mm Hg should be treated aggressively; even a partial response is likely to reduce the morbidity associated with this condition

(B) patients 35 years or younger who have normal diastolic blood pressure but a systolic blood pressure in excess of 150 mm Hg should have their diastolic blood pressure checked every 4 months

(C) a significant reduction in the incidence of cardiovascular and cerebrovascular disease may be expected if a patient with a constant diastolic blood pressure between 90 and 104 mm Hg has blood pressure returned to a normal level

(D) more than 700 out of every 1000 diabetics who are 45 years old and have left ventricular hypertrophy, a cholesterol level in excess of 335 mg/dl, and systemic blood pressure of 195 mm Hg or greater will have serious cardiovascular disease within 8 years

(E) systolic blood pressure above 160 mm Hg in patients above 60 years of age should be treated even if the diastolic blood pressure is normal

204. All the following statements concerning thrombolytic therapy in acute myocardial infarction are correct EXCEPT

(A) urokinase is less antigenic than streptokinase

(B) tissue-type plasminogen activator (t-PA) does not create a lytic state

(C) intravenous streptokinase is at least as effective as intracoronary streptokinase in thrombus dissolution

(D) uncontrolled hypertension is a contraindication to thrombolytic therapy

(E) side effects requiring discontinuation of therapy occur in 15 percent of patients treated with streptokinase

205. A 75-year-old woman suffering from an acute anterior wall myocardial infarction is admitted to a coronary care unit. An ECG monitor strip, obtained 6 hours after admission, discloses the rhythm illustrated below. This rhythm probably represents

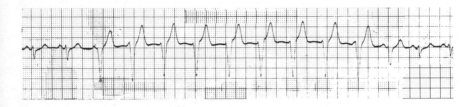

(A) rate-dependent left bundle branch block
(B) rate-dependent right bundle branch block
(C) complete heart block
(D) accelerated idioventricular rhythm
(E) junctional rhythm

---

206. Each of the following statements regarding ventricular aneurysms is true EXCEPT that

(A) they should be suspected in the presence of a persistent ST-segment elevation following a myocardial infarction
(B) they are more common with anterior than inferior wall myocardial infarctions
(C) affected patients have an increased risk of cardiac rupture
(D) recurrent arterial emboli may be the presenting sign
(E) the diagnosis may be suggested by the x-ray finding of calcium in the cardiac border

207. Idiopathic hypertrophic subaortic stenosis is characterized by all the following statements EXCEPT that

(A) the carotid pulse of affected patients reveals a slow upstroke
(B) the associated murmur increases in a standing position
(C) a prominent fourth heart sound frequently occurs
(D) mitral regurgitation is present in 50 percent of affected patients
(E) propranolol is useful for treating affected patients who have dyspnea or light-headedness

208. The rhythm strip displayed below reveals normal sinus rhythm with

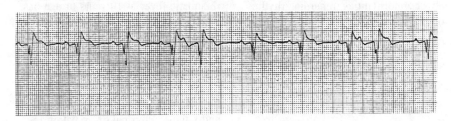

(A) periods of atrioventricular dissociation
(B) periods of Wenckebach atrioventricular block
(C) atrial premature contractions
(D) junctional premature contractions
(E) ventricular premature contractions

209. The rhythm strip (lead II) shown below was obtained from a patient who had severe obstructive lung disease. The strip most closely depicts which of the following arrhythmias?

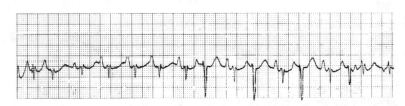

(A) Atrial flutter with varying atrioventricular block
(B) Sinus tachycardia with premature atrial contractions
(C) Sinus tachycardia with premature ventricular contractions
(D) Atrioventricular dissociation
(E) Multifocal atrial tachycardia

210. All the following statements about abnormalities in cardiac rhythm or rate are true EXCEPT that

(A) the treatment of sinus bradycardia (a rate less than 60/min) following myocardial infarction is mandatory if an affected patient is experiencing ventricular premature beats occurring at a rate of three or more per minute
(B) ventricular tachycardia occurring after myocardial infarction can be initially treated with lidocaine if an affected patient is not in heart failure
(C) digoxin is not contraindicated in the management of cardiac failure associated with ventricular tachycardia
(D) anticoagulation therapy is of little use in patients with atrial fibrillation who suffer thromboemboli following elective reversion to sinus rhythm
(E) quinidine should never be used in patients with atrial flutter without the prior or concomitant administration of digoxin or propranolol

211. A syphilitic aneurysm of the aorta is most likely to occur at which of the following sites?

(A) Ascending aorta
(B) Aortic arch
(C) Descending thoracic aorta
(D) Abdominal aorta
(E) Bifurcation of the iliac arteries

212. A 40-year-old woman who had rheumatic fever at 10 years of age has had a heart murmur for the past 15 years. Over the past 3 years she has noted progressive dyspnea on exertion, orthopnea, and fatigue. She is presently unable to do even light housework without developing shortness of breath and fatigue. Physical examination reveals a loud first heart sound and opening snap that is very close to the second heart sound. There is a grade III/VI middiastolic rumble at the cardiac apex with presystolic accentuation. Cardiac catheterization reveals pure mitral stenosis with a calculated valve area of 0.8 cm². No mitral regurgitation is present. Management of this patient should consist of

(A) penicillin prophylaxis
(B) administration of anticoagulants
(C) digitalization
(D) mitral valve commissurotomy
(E) mitral valve replacement

213. An 18-year-old man is involved in a street fight during which he sustains a severe knife wound to the chest. As a consequence of this injury, bleeding occurs into his pericardial cavity. He is placed on broad-spectrum antibiotic coverage that includes ampicillin and gentamicin. He makes a good recovery over the following month but 3 months after the incident he suddenly becomes ill with a fever of 39.6°C (103.3°F). The symptoms and signs consist of pericarditis, pleuritis, and pneumonitis. In the 3 days that follow, the patient develops arthralgias, pericardial effusion, and leukocytosis. The most likely diagnosis of this condition is

(A) serum sickness induced by ampicillin
(B) rheumatoid arthritis
(C) Dressler's syndrome
(D) acute idiopathic pericarditis
(E) acute bacterial endocarditis

214. A 65-year-old man complains of chest pain, shortness of breath, and syncope. He has a long history of a heart murmur but was asymptomatic until 1 year ago when he noted retrosternal chest pain occurring on exertion but relieved by rest. The chest pains have continued, and he has noted exertional dyspnea for the past several months. On two occasions following heavy exertion, the patient passed out for several seconds. Physical examination reveals a blood pressure of 110/80 mm Hg and pulse of 50/minute. The carotid upstroke is markedly delayed; there is a palpable systolic thrill. Lung fields reveal rales in both bases. The point of maximum intensity is in the fifth intercostal space, midclavicular line. There is a prominent left ventricular heave. The first heart sound is soft and aortic closure is decreased. A grade IV/VI harsh, late-peaking systolic murmur is heard over the aortic area. Third and fourth heart sounds are present at the apex. The electrocardiogram reveals sinus bradycardia and left ventricular hypertrophy. The chest x-ray shows cardiomegaly with congestive heart failure. The most appropriate measure in the management of this patient would be

(A) stress testing
(B) cardiac catheterization
(C) oral propranolol and long-acting nitrates
(D) diuretics and digitalis
(E) a permanent pacemaker

215. A 45-year-old asymptomatic airline pilot is subjected to exercise-induced cardiac stress tests as part of a biannual physical examination. At the end of a quite strenuous exercise test (heart rate greater than 150/minute), he develops a 3-mm ST-segment depression in leads V_1 to V_4. However, he has no pain or other symptoms. There is no family history of early ischemic heart disease or hypertension and the patient has normal lipid studies. The advice you should give to this patient would be which of the following?

(A) The risk of sudden myocardial ischemia is too high to allow you to continue as a commercial pilot
(B) You should have coronary angiography to determine the condition of your coronary vessels
(C) You should have the test repeated in a month; if it is still positive, you should stop flying and have coronary angiography
(D) You can continue to fly safely only if you receive anticoagulants and take long-acting drugs to dilate your coronary blood vessels
(E) Your electrocardiographic changes are without significance and correlate poorly with sudden death and other complications of heart disease

216. A 23-year-old woman with no previous history of cardiac disease develops symptoms and signs of acute bacterial endocarditis with mitral incompetence 1 week after an abortion. *Streptococcus faecalis* is grown in blood cultures. The most appropriate treatment for this patient would be

(A) mitral valve replacement followed by 6 weeks of antibiotic therapy
(B) parenteral administration of ampicillin, 12 g daily for 4 weeks
(C) parenteral administration of penicillin G, 24 million units per day for 6 weeks
(D) parenteral administration of penicillin G, 24 million units per day, and gentamicin, 4 mg/kg daily for 4 weeks
(E) parenteral administration of vancomycin, 1 g daily for 4 weeks, with streptomycin, 1 g daily added to the protocol for the first 2 weeks

DIRECTIONS: Each question below contains four suggested responses of which **one or more** is correct. Select

A	if	**1, 2, and 3**	are correct
B	if	**1 and 3**	are correct
C	if	**2 and 4**	are correct
D	if	**4**	is correct
E	if	**1, 2, 3, and 4**	are correct

217. A 54-year old man with a history of viral pericarditis is found on physical examination to have hepatomegaly and distended neck veins; chest x-rays reveal calcification of the pericardium. Correct statements concerning this patient's condition include which of the following?

(1) Episodes of acute pulmonary edema punctuate the clinical course

(2) It may be complicated by a protein-losing gastroenteropathy

(3) A paradoxical pulse is an uncommon finding

(4) Echocardiography demonstrates paradoxical septal motion

218. Correct statements concerning renovascular hypertension include which of the following?

(1) The presence of grade 3 or 4 hypertensive retinopathy increases the likelihood of renovascular hypertension

(2) Measuring peripheral vein renin is useful in detecting renovascular hypertension

(3) The onset of hypertension usually occurs before age 35 in patients with fibrous dysplasia of the renal artery

(4) An abdominal bruit is a rare finding in patients with fibrous dysplasia of the renal artery

219. A patient with a congenital bicuspid valve develops auscultatory evidence of aortic regurgitation. True statements regarding this condition include which of the following?

(1) Angina pectoris in the absence of coronary artery disease is uncommon

(2) Syncope in the absence of dysrhythmia rarely, if ever, occurs

(3) Prophylaxis against bacterial endocarditis is indicated for surgical instrumentation of the genitourinary tract

(4) Asymptomatic patients who show evidence by echocardiography of left ventricular dysfunction at rest should be advised to have surgery

220. When fluid in the pericardial space exceeds the 20 ml of volume normally present, cardiac tamponade may ensue. Correct statements concerning this clinical entity include which of the following?

(1) Loss of the y descent and accentuation of the x descent are seen on the right atrial pressure waveform

(2) A large inspiratory fall in arterial systolic pressure is not associated with cardiac tamponade

(3) Myocardial ischemia may result from compression of epicardial vessels

(4) An inspiratory increase in jugular venous pressure (Kussmaul's sign) is characteristic

DIRECTIONS: Each group of questions below consists of lettered headings followed by a set of numbered items. For each numbered item select the **one** lettered heading with which it is **most** closely associated. Each lettered heading may be used **once, more than once, or not at all.**

Questions 221–223

For each cardiac disorder below, select the clinical finding with which it is most closely associated.

(A) Sharp y descent in jugular pulse tracing
(B) Middiastolic rumble at apex
(C) Large v waves in jugular pulse tracing
(D) Slow y descent in jugular pulse tracing
(E) Prominent c waves in jugular pulse tracing

221. Tricuspid stenosis

222. Aortic regurgitation

223. Constrictive pericarditis

Questions 224–227

Match the agents below with associated side effects.

(A) Increased triglyceride levels
(B) Volume retention
(C) Lupuslike syndrome
(D) Nephrotic syndrome
(E) Gynecomastia

224. Captopril

225. Hydralazine

226. Propranolol

227. Minoxidil

Questions 228–231

For each electrolyte abnormality below, select the electrocardiographic picture with which it is most commonly associated.

(A) No known electrocardiographic abnormalities
(B) Prolonged Q-T interval
(C) Short Q-T interval
(D) Widened QRS complex
(E) Prominent U waves

228. Hypokalemia

229. Hyperkalemia

230. Hypocalcemia

231. Hyponatremia

Questions 232–236

A normal jugular venous pulse wave in relation to first and second heart sounds is displayed below. For each cardiac phenomenon described, select the segment of the venous pulse wave with which it is most likely to be associated.

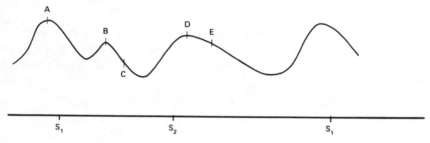

232. Atrial contraction

233. Filling of right atrium while tricuspid valve is closed

234. Opening of tricuspid valve

235. Bulging of tricuspid valve into right atrium

236. S_4 gallop

Questions 237–239

Match the following.

(A) Bronchiectasis
(B) Coarctation of the aorta
(C) Ventricular septal defect
(D) Homocystinuria
(E) None of the above

237. Dextrocardia

238. Aortic and pulmonary artery dilatation

239. Hyperextensible joints

Cardiology
Answers

178. The answer is D. *(Braunwald, ed 11. p 902. Thomas, p 228.)* The physiological adaptation of the cardiovascular system to strenuous exercise is being increasingly studied as not only professional athletes but the general public become more and more interested in maximizing physical performance. Perhaps the most notable cardiovascular change involves the lowering of the pulse rate as an increased stroke volume markedly increases the efficiency of each cardiac contraction. To achieve the maximum possible improvement in cardiac performance regular isotonic exercise is needed. Various studies have demonstrated that this result is achieved by physical activity three to five times a week at 60 to 90 percent of maximal heart rate for at least 15 minutes but no longer than 60 minutes. As oxygen consumption relates directly to the amount of muscular work performed, the capacity to deliver oxygen efficiently to exercising muscles, thus avoiding anaerobic metabolism, which of necessity limits the duration of exercise, is a sure measure of successful adaptive cardiovascular changes. This can be measured as the $V_{O_{2max}}$. As the work load increases, even well-trained muscles demand more and more oxygen. The ability to deliver oxygen more efficiently to the tissues involves both central (cardiac) adaptation, as well as peripheral (muscular) change. Measuring the difference between the arterial and venous oxygen in an exercising limb gives one a good measurement of the efficiency of oxygen extraction. The $V_{O_{2max}}$ is affected by age such that the average person of 60 can perform only 66 percent of the work capacity of a person of 20 years. Healthy but sedentary people who begin exercising can expect a 30 to 40 percent improvement in their $V_{O_{2max}}$. Of interest, putting anyone to bed rest for 3 to 4 weeks results in a 20 to 25 percent decrease in $V_{O_{2max}}$. The importance of peripheral adaptive changes can be noted from studies in which only the leg muscles are involved in vigorous training exercises. Oxygen exchange in these muscles will become markedly more efficient while nonexercised muscle groups will show no significant change.

179. The answer is E. *(Braunwald, ed 11. pp 1102–1105. Hurst, ed 6. pp 590–603, 658–659, 662–667, 1099–1103.)* In the patient presented in the question, the absence of a history of heart murmur makes congenital heart disease an unlikely diagnosis. The rapid onset of the symptoms described makes primary pulmonary hypertension the most likely cause. While its cause is unknown, the basic pathology of this disease involves thickening of the walls of the pulmonary arterioles resulting in progressive resistance to blood flow through the lungs. As the disease progresses, pulmonary blood flow and cardiac output are reduced and show little increase during exertion. Primary pulmonary hypertension tends to have a peak incidence in young women. Death usually occurs within 4 to 5 years after onset of symptoms. Affected patients characteristically have the symptom complex and physical findings described in the question. Systolic ejection murmurs in the pulmonic area result from ejection of blood into a proximally dilated pulmonary artery. Holosystolic murmurs at the lower left sternal border probably represent tricuspid insufficiency from right ventricular enlargement. Dilatation of the proximal portion of the pulmonary arteries, with decreased blood flow to the outer third of the lung fields, is a further indication of pulmonary hypertension.

180. The answer is E. *(Meltzer, Ann Intern Med 104:689–698, 1986.)* With the advent of two-dimensional echocardiography, many studies have been done to determine the natural history of cardiac thrombi and their risk of embolization. These studies have determined that anticoagulation therapy is warranted in patients with myocardial infarctions associated with congestive heart failure regardless of infarct location and in patients with anterior myocardial infarctions who have echocardiographically demonstrated left ventricular thrombi. Interestingly, while thrombi occur frequently in left ventricular aneurysms, they embolize infrequently and antithrombotic therapy is therefore not indicated. This is in contradistinction to patients with idiopathic dilated cardiomyopathy who have high rates of embolization and in whom anticoagulation therapy is recommended.

181. The answer is D. *(Hurst, ed 6. pp 464–465, 480.)* Type I AV block, the more common of the two forms of second-degree AV block, is characterized by the following: (1) after progressive lengthening of the P-R interval, the final P wave is not followed by a QRS complex, (2) the increment by which the P-R interval increases progressively decreases, and (3) the R-R interval containing the dropped beat is less than two times the shortest preceding R-R interval. Type I AV block is due to a conduction delay within the AV node. Progression to complete AV block is unusual and the rhythm is generally benign.

182. The answer is E. *(Hurst, ed 6. pp 1120–1125.)* Cor pulmonale is characterized by the presence of pulmonary hypertension and consequent right ventricular dysfunction. Its causes include diseases leading to hypoxic vasoconstriction, as in cystic fibrosis; occlusion of the pulmonary vasculature, as in pulmonary thromboembolism; and parenchymal destruction, as in sarcoidosis. The right ventricle, in the presence of a chronic increase in afterload, becomes hypertrophic, dilates, and fails. The electrocardiographic findings, as illustrated in the question, include tall, peaked P waves in leads II, III, and aVF, which indicate right atrial enlargement; tall R waves in leads V_1 to V_3 and a deep S wave in V_6 with associated ST-T wave changes, which indicate right ventricular hypertrophy; and right axis deviation. Right bundle branch block occurs in 15 percent of patients.

183. The answer is C. *(Braunwald, ed 11. p 934. Somberg, Am Heart J 111:1162–1176, 1986.)* Torsade de pointes is a rapid ventricular tachycardia characterized by unusual QRS complexes whose axes shift back and forth around the baseline. It occurs most commonly in patients who have prolonged Q-T intervals during sinus rhythm. Indeed, any influence that prolongs the Q-T interval, such as quinidine, procainamide, tricyclic antidepressants, phenothiazines, hypokalemia, or hypocalcemia, or congenital Q-T prolongation may cause torsade. This rhythm is clinically important because it may degenerate to ventricular fibrillation, and it should not be treated with Q-T–lengthening antiarrhythmics. Emergent therapy may include either ventricular pacing or isoproterenol infusion along with correction of the underlying abnormality in the acquired forms or with the addition of drugs that shorten the Q-T interval, such as phenytoin and beta blockers, in the congenital varieties.

184. The answer is B. *(Hein, Am J Med 64:27–33, 1978.)* Diagnosis of the site of origin of a tachycardia with a widened QRS complex is critical both prognostically and therapeutically. Several criteria have been advanced on the differentiation between a supraventricular and a ventricular origin of wide QRS complexes during tachycardia based on reviews of ECGs and concomitant His-bundle electrography: (1) Aberrant conduction is favored in the presence of right bundle branch block–shaped QRS complexes at a frequency above 170/min. (2) AV dissociation during tachycardia favors a ventricular origin. (3) Ventricular tachycardia is usually a regular rhythm; however, alternation of the R-R interval during tachycardia may occur in both ventricular and supraventricular tachycardias. (4) A QRS width of greater than 0.14 sec favors a ventricular focus, as does left axis deviation in the frontal plane. (5) A ventricular origin is also favored in the finding of mono- or biphasic right bundle branch block–shaped QRS complexes in lead V_1. Triphasic right bundle branch block–shaped QRS complexes in lead V_1 are not helpful as they are found in both supraventricular and ventricular tachycardia.

185. The answer is E. *(Braunwald, ed 11. pp 921–922. Mandel, ed 2. pp 241–253.)* The rhythm strip exhibited both in the question and below reveals a P wave before the first QRS complex, with a short P-R interval. The P waves then move into the QRS complexes until the end of the strip where a P wave is again seen preceding a QRS complex. The P-R intervals and the QRS intervals are almost identical. This strip reveals atrioventricular (AV) dissociation in which the atria are being depolarized by the sinus node and the ventricles are being depolarized by a junctional or AV nodal focus. This particular example of AV dissociation is termed "isorhythmic dissociation" since the rates of atria and ventricles are almost equal. The preferred meaning of AV dissociation implies two separate pacemakers, with the lower focus faster in rate than the higher focus. This situation differs from complete heart block, in which the rate of the lower focus is slower than the higher, since it is an escape rhythm. In AV dissociation, the lower focus is firing faster than the higher because of increased automaticity and thus controlling the ventricles only because it is firing faster than the sinus node. AV dissociation is commonly associated with digitalis toxicity, inferior wall myocardial infarction, and hypokalemia.

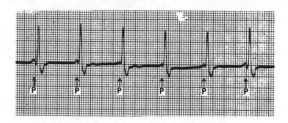

186. The answer is C. *(Braunwald, ed 11. pp 1004–1005.)* Myxomas are histologically benign and account for up to one-half of all cases of primary cardiac tumors. Because they are most commonly located in the left atrium and are pedunculated, they are particularly prone to causing mitral stenosis as a result of a ball-valve effect and mitral regurgitation due to trauma to the mitral leaflets. Noncardiac manifestations of myxomas include fever, weight loss, arthralgia, Raynaud's phenomenon, and anemia. Surgical excision is curative. Cardiac sarcomas are the most common malignant primary cardiac tumor and are uniformly rapidly fatal.

187. The answer is D. *(Braunwald, ed 11. pp 1019–1022.)* To date, reduction of excessive cardiovascular morbidity has been demonstrated clearly only in patients whose diastolic pressures had exceeded 105 mm Hg. There is a growing consensus among cardiologists, however, that the diastolic pressure should be kept at, or below, 90 mm Hg. Excellent evidence now suggests that high density lipoproteins, which can absorb 20 percent of the total plasma cholesterol, protect against the development of atherosclerosis and, therefore, should be considered to be antirisk factors. A decrease in cigarette smoking and the undertaking of regular exercise both raise the circulating level of high density lipoproteins. Epidemiological studies have conclusively demonstrated the benefit of stopping cigarette smoking, as well as the dangers of smoking. Elevations in systolic blood pressure, though less damaging than elevations in diastolic blood pressure, are definitely associated with an increased risk of cardiovascular disease.

188. The answer is A. *(Braunwald, ed 11. pp 962–963.)* The fundamental defect in mitral valve prolapse is an abnormality of the valve's connective tissue with secondary proliferation of myxomatous tissue. The redundant leaflet or leaflets prolapse toward the left atrium in systole resulting in the auscultated click and murmur and characteristic echocardiographic findings. Any maneuver that reduces left ventricular size, such as standing and Valsalva, allows the click and murmur to occur earlier in systole; conversely, those maneuvers that increase left ventricular size, such as squatting and propranolol administration, delay the onset of the click and murmur. While most patients with mitral valve prolapse have a benign prognosis, a small percentage die suddenly. Antibiotic prophylaxis to prevent endocarditis is recommended for those with typical auscultatory findings.

189. The answer is E. *(Hurst, ed 6. pp 1624–1635.)* Three calcium channel blockers—nifedipine, verapamil, and diltiazem—are used in treating such diverse diseases as hypertension, cardiac arrhythmias, angina pectoris, and idiopathic hypertrophic subaortic stenosis. All three drugs have a coronary vasodilator effect. Only verapamil, however, is capable of suppressing most cases of supraventricular tachycardia, atrial flutter, and fibrillation; it is not effective in ventricular arrhythmias and in converting atrial fibrillation to normal sinus rhythm. Because these drugs display negative inotropic effects, they should be used with caution in patients with depressed left ventricular function. Verapamil, and to a lesser extent nifedipine, both increase serum digoxin levels with a steady state reached within 1 to 4 weeks of combined administration.

190. The answer is C. *(Braunwald, ed 11. pp 1037–1038.)* Seventy-five percent of aortic aneurysms occur in the abdominal aorta just below the renal arteries. The majority of such aneurysms occur in men; the mean age of occurrence is 60. More than half the cases are associated with elevations in blood pressure. Most commonly the diagnosis is made on routine physical examination. Ultrasound is the noninvasive investigation of choice and will delineate the mass and provide the diameter of the aneurysm and the thickness of its walls. Small-diameter aneurysms (less than 6 cm) present a 15 to 20 percent chance of rupture. However, as fatalities associated with this complication approximate 50 percent and the operative mortality for elective procedures of small-diameter aneurysms is only 5 percent, it is prudent to recommend surgery for affected patients. Five-year survival rates for patients with aortic aneurysms without cardiovascular disease is 50 percent; with cardiovascular disease it is only 20 percent. In the presence of other cardiovascular disease, small-diameter aneurysms may be followed by serial ultrasound examinations. Risk associated with surgery in these patients is substantial. Information on changes in the aneurysm provided by ultrasound examinations would be useful in making a decision on the necessity of surgery.

191. The answer is C. *(Braunwald, ed 11. pp 931–932. Mandel, ed 2. pp 261–263.)* The electrocardiogram presented in the question demonstrates an acute inferior wall myocardial infarction with ST-segment elevation in leads II, III, and aVF. A significant Q wave is present in lead III. The ST-segment depressions seen in the majority of the other leads are probably reciprocal changes to the ST-segment elevations mentioned. The ST-segment elevation of acute pericarditis, however, is not accompanied by reciprocal changes. Close examination of the tracing reveals P waves following each QRS complex. Whether the P wave precedes, is buried within, or follows the QRS complex in a nodal rhythm or nodal tachycardia depends upon the location of the ectopic focus in the atrioventricular (AV) node and the rates of antegrade and retrograde conduction. In this example, the ectopic focus in the AV node reaches the ventricle just before it reaches the atrium, resulting in the P wave following the QRS complex. Nodal tachycardia is diagnosed when the rate of the pacemaker in the AV node exceeds 60 per minute. Common causes of this arrhythmia are inferior wall myocardial infarction, digitalis intoxication, and myocarditis.

192. The answer is C. *(Braunwald, ed 11. p 927. Mandel, ed 2. pp 228–230.)* The rhythm strip exhibited in the question reveals atrial flutter with 4:1 atrioventricular (AV) block. Atrial flutter is characterized by an atrial rate of 280 to 320 per minute; the electrocardiogram typically reveals a sawtooth baseline configuration due to the flutter waves. In the strip presented, every fourth atrial depolarization is conducted through the AV node, resulting in a ventricular rate of 75 per minute.

193. The answer is B. *(Braunwald, ed 11. pp 1007, 1586.)* Tumors producing the carcinoid syndrome are slowly growing neoplasms arising from the gastrointestinal tract or derivatives of the embryonic foregut, testes, and ovaries. Their clinical features include cutaneous flushing, telangiectasis, intestinal hypermotility, bronchospasm, and evidence of valvular heart disease. The right side of the heart is more commonly involved than the left and there is a tendency of developing tricuspid regurgitation and pulmonic stenosis with consequent right-sided heart failure. The morbidity from these tumors results largely from their variable expression of serotonin, histamine, substance P, and bradykinin. While no effective antitumor regimen exists, therapy using histamine and serotonin antagonists may be helpful.

194. The answer is C. *(Braunwald, ed 11. pp 951–956.)* Streptococcal antibody titers rise so consistently after streptococcal infection that they can be relied upon to help rule out respiratory tract infections caused by other organisms. Without serological evidence of a recent streptococcal infection, one should hesitate to make a diagnosis of rheumatic fever. However, two exceptions should be kept in mind. Occasionally, symptoms that are suggestive of acute rheumatic fever may not develop for as long as 2 months after the initial infectious episode. This is particularly the case in patients with Sydenham's chorea. As the antistreptococcal titers will have peaked before this period, the declining levels may be misleading. The situation is even more difficult in patients who have no other symptoms of rheumatic fever besides a pancarditis. In such cases, it may be several months after the acute infection before a diagnosis is made. Such patients may have low antibody titers when seen initially.

195. The answer is D. *(Braunwald, ed 11. pp 879–880. Mandel, ed 2. pp 102–105.)* The electrocardiogram shown in the question reveals an evolving anteroseptal myocardial infarction. There is ST-segment elevation in leads V_1 to V_3. Right bundle branch block (RBBB) is present with QRS duration of 0.12 second and terminal, wide S waves in leads I, aVL, and V_8. The classic rSR' of RBBB is not seen since the initial r wave in V_1 has been replaced with a Q wave as a result of the anterior infarction. The electrocardiogram also reveals marked left axis deviation consistent with a left anterior hemiblock. Since both the right bundle and the anterior division of the left bundle are damaged as a result of the infarction, conduction to the ventricles is dependent solely on the posterior division of the left bundle. In the presence of an acute anteroseptal myocardial infarction, temporary transvenous pacing is indicated for the patient involved as a prophylactic measure to avert complete heart block.

196. The answer is C. *(Braunwald, ed 11. pp 943–945. Hoeprich, ed 3. p 1175.)* Atrial septal defects are rarely involved in endocarditis probably because there is no large pressure gradient across the defect. Significant pressure gradients created by other congenital cardiac lesions result in turbulence, which appears to be one of the predisposing factors for the deposition of fibrin and bacteria.

197. The answer is A. *(Braunwald, ed 11. pp 989–991. Mandel, ed 2. pp 303–308.)* The first part of the rhythm strip shown in the question demonstrates Mobitz II atrioventricular (AV) block with every other P wave conducted to the ventricles. A ventricular premature contraction is then noted, followed by P waves without any QRS complexes. There is complete lack of conduction of the atrial impulses and, furthermore, a lack of any subsidiary pacemaker to maintain cardiac rhythm. The most appropriate immediate therapy for this conduction problem would be cardiopulmonary resuscitation and infusion of isoproterenol. Isoproterenol increases automaticity of cardiac pacemakers and thus may provoke a subsidiary pacemaker to start firing. Atropine might be useful except that the presence of Mobitz II block and wide QRS complexes suggests disease below the AV node, where atropine exerts little effect on subsidiary pacemakers. Intracardiac epinephrine should be used only as a last resort.

198. The answer is A. *(Forrester, N Engl J Med 205:1356–1360, 1976.)* The Swan-Ganz pulmonary artery catheter provides an accurate bedside means of determining left ventricular filling pressures. The catheter is passed through a vein to the heart where it is placed in a pulmonary artery. When the balloon at the tip is inflated, the catheter records pulmonary capillary pressure, which is equivalent to left atrial pressure and, in the absence of mitral stenosis, to left ventricular diastolic pressure. The level of pulmonary capillary pressure correlates with left ventricular volume. Normal pulmonary capillary pressure is 5 to 12 mm Hg. Levels above 18 to 20 mm Hg are associated with signs of congestive heart failure. On admission to the hospital, the patient presented in the question had bibasilar rales, which probably resulted from his cigarette smoking, since an S_3 gallop, which would have suggested congestive failure, was not heard. His postdiuretic pulmonary capillary pressure of 4 mm Hg is low and indicates hypovolemia. Appropriate therapy for this patient would be to administer intravenous fluids to bring his pulmonary capillary pressures up to at least 10 to 12 mm Hg.

199. The answer is D. *(Braunwald, ed 11. p 992. Hurst, ed 6. pp 393–394, 983–984.)* The most likely diagnoses in any patient suffering acute myocardial infarction who develops severe congestive failure and a new murmur are ventricular septal defect (VSD) and papillary muscle dysfunction (PMD). While both VSD and PMD can occur with an anteroseptal infarction, VSD is the more common. The murmur of acquired VSD following infarction tends to be maximal at the lower sternal border and may be associated with a thrill. Mitral regurgitation due to PMD is usually maximal at the apex. However, it is sometimes very difficult to determine exactly which defect is present. Rupture of a papillary muscle is a catastrophic event associated with shock and intractable pulmonary edema. The hypoxemia exhibited by the patient presented in the question, while suggestive of pulmonary embolism, is compatible with severe congestive failure alone.

200. The answer is B. *(Hurst, ed 6. pp 172–173.)* Normally, the second heart sound (S_2) is composed of aortic closure followed by pulmonic closure. Because inspiration increases blood return to the right side of the heart, pulmonic closure is delayed resulting in normal splitting of S_2 during inspiration. Paradoxical splitting of S_2, however, refers to a splitting of S_2 that is narrowed instead of widened with inspiration consequent to a delayed aortic closure. Paradoxical splitting can result from any electrical or mechanical event that delays left ventricular systole. Thus, aortic stenosis and hypertension, which increase resistance to systolic ejection of blood, delay closure of the aortic valve. Acute ischemia from angina or acute myocardial infarction also can delay ejection of blood from the left ventricle. The most common cause of paradoxical splitting—left bundle branch block—delays electrical activation of the left ventricle. Right bundle branch block results in a wide splitting of S_2 that widens further during inspiration.

201. The answer is D. *(Braunwald, ed 11. pp 913–914.)* Many compensatory changes occur in the heart and vascular bed of patients experiencing heart failure. One such mechanism involves the active constriction of peripheral vessels. This constriction results in persistent tension in the myocardium of the left ventricle (left ventricular afterload). If cardiac function is already impaired, this additional factor may significantly worsen the situation by reducing cardiac output and further increasing myocardial consumption of oxygen. A major advance in the treatment of severe heart failure has been the development of drugs that can dilate the peripheral vessels, thus reducing vessel wall obstruction to left ventricular ejection. The various vasodilators that are available have different hemodynamic effects, loci, and durations of action. The modes of administration also differ. The ideal vasodilating drug would be administered orally and have a sustained effect for at least 6 hours. Some vasodilators, such as the alpha-adrenergic blocking agents and hydralazine, affect the arterial bed, while others, such as nitroglycerin, only affect resistance in the venous circulation. Hydralazine is an ideal choice for the patient who needs long-term treatment and vasodilation of the arterial circulation. Nitroglycerin has a short-lived effect on the venous system. Isosorbide dinitrate affects the same vessels but is longer-acting than nitroglycerin. Phentolamine, which works on arterial beds, lasts for minutes only and must be given by continuous intravenous infusion. The same objections apply to trimethaphan. Nitroprusside, which affects both venous and arterial beds, is ideal for the management of acute heart failure. It is effective for only minutes, however, and must be given by continuous intravenous infusion.

202.   The answer is B. *(Braunwald, ed 11. p 948.)* Coarctation of the aorta consists of a region of narrowed aorta; 95 percent of these lesions occur just distal to the left subclavian artery. Because of decreased blood flow to the lower extremities, affected patients may complain of leg fatigue or pain on exertion. A congenital bicuspid aortic valve occurs concomitantly with coarctation in approximately 50 percent of such people. Symptoms of congestive heart failure are common in infants who have coarctation and usually appear in the first months of life. Patients afflicted with Turner's syndrome have a high incidence of aortic coarctation.

203.   The answer is B. *(Braunwald, ed 11. pp 1024–1036.)* The study data obtained from the 18-year prospective study in Framingham, Massachusetts, strongly suggest that cardiovascular disease is related to hypertension, serum cholesterol level, cigarette smoking, glucose intolerance, and electrocardiographic evidence of hypertrophy of the left ventricle. Although the need to reduce the blood pressure of patients with diastolic levels above 105 mm Hg is well established, the need to aggressively treat patients whose blood pressure falls between the 90 to 104 mm Hg range has remained controversial. Several clinical trials in different parts of the world have demonstrated significant benefits from such an approach. Long-term follow-up studies show significant reductions in the development of cerebrovascular accidents, congestive cardiac failure, myocardial infarction, and aortic dissection. Data based on the Framingham study reveal the worst-case situation. A 45-year-old man with a high systolic pressure, diabetes, a high level serum cholesterol, and a left ventricle already enlarged has a more than 70 percent chance of suffering from severe cardiovascular disease within an 8-year period. The treatment of systolic blood pressure, when diastolic levels are normal, is also important. While long-term studies to show the benefit of the reduction of systolic blood pressure have not as yet been concluded, what data are available suggest that one is being very conservative in strongly recommending that systolic blood pressure above 160 mm Hg should be treated in patients who are over 60 years of age. In patients who are younger than 35 years of age, systolic blood pressure that persistently lies above 140 mm Hg should be controlled. Between the ages of 35 and 60, current recommendations call for the treatment of systolic blood pressure greater than 150 mm Hg.

204. The answer is E. *(Rackley, pp 39–49.)* In recent years, attempts at reducing myocardial necrosis in patients with acute myocardial infarction have included intraaortic balloon counterpulsation; administration of beta blockers, calcium channel blockers, and nitrates; and insulin-glucose-phosphate infusions. Thrombolytic therapy, involving either streptokinase (STK), urokinase (UK), or t-Pa is now undergoing clinical trials. STK, a product of group C beta-hemolytic streptococci, activates the fibrinolytic system by combining with plasminogen; this complex then converts uncomplexed plasminogen to plasmin, which in turn causes thrombus dissolution. Significant side effects are distinctly uncommon. UK also activates the fibrinolytic system but through direct activation of plasminogen. Because it is less antigenic than streptokinase, the risk of inactivation owing to previous exposure is not as great. t-PA is a naturally occurring protease that binds to fibrinogen, and it is this complex that converts plasminogen to plasmin. Because plasminogen is converted to plasmin at the surface of the clot and not diffusely in the circulation, a lytic state is not created. While studies have shown high rates of successful coronary reperfusion, the long-term ramifications are still undetermined.

205. The answer is D. *(Braunwald, ed 11. p 934. Hurst, ed 6. p 976.)* The ECG strip presented in the question demonstrates normal sinus rhythm with a period of accelerated idioventricular rhythm (AIVR). AIVR may arise from increased automaticity or occur as an escape rhythm and usually is seen either after acute myocardial infarction or in digitalis intoxication. On the ECG, the rate of the AIVR is slightly faster than that of the first two sinus beats. Beats numbered 3 and 12 represent fusion beats since the QRS configuration is intermediate between that of the sinus beats and those of AIVR. Characteristics of this arrhythmia are the wide, bizarre complexes resembling premature ventricular contractions, the presence of fusion beats, and a rate of 55 to 125/minute. Rate-dependent left or right bundle branch block is accompanied by widening of the QRS complex but each complex is preceded by a constant P-R interval. In complete heart block, P waves are independent of the QRS complexes and occur at a rate faster than the QRS complexes. Junctional rhythms most commonly occur at rates of 40 to 60/minute and the QRS complexes are usually normal in configuration.

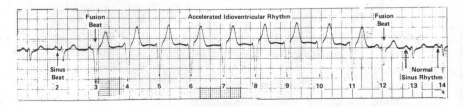

206. The answer is C. *(Hurst, ed 6. pp 847–850, 986–987, 1673.)* The formation of a ventricular aneurysm is a late complication of myocardial infarction and the diagnosis is usually first suggested by the presence of persistent ST-segment elevation several months after the infarction. Patients who have an aneurysm may present with arterial emboli, recurrent ventricular arrhythmias, or intractable congestive heart failure. Rupture is extremely unlikely unless there is a reinfarction over the same involved area of the ventricle. The chest x-ray occasionally reveals calcium in the wall of the aneurysm or in a mural thrombus in the middle of the aneurysm. Once confirmed by angiography, the aneurysm may be resected.

207. The answer is A. *(Braunwald, ed 11. pp 1002–1003.)* Idiopathic hypertrophic subaortic stenosis (IHSS) is characterized by thickening of the muscular interventricular septum resulting in obstruction to left ventricular ejection of blood during ventricular systole. The typical murmur is a systolic ejection murmur along the left sternal border. Any maneuver that increases left ventricular volume will decrease the obstruction and murmur. Conversely, standing, which causes venous pooling in the lower extremities, will decrease ventricular volume and thus cause the obstruction and murmur to increase. The arterial pulse has a typical brisk upstroke and may display two palpable peaks in the pulse wave. A loud fourth heart sound is common and results from the atrium attempting to eject blood into a thick, noncompliant ventricle. The thick septum associated with IHSS, by displacing the anterior leaflet of the mitral valve, causes mitral regurgitation in 50 percent of affected patients. Propranolol, by decreasing the contractility of the heart, may relieve the obstruction to left ventricular ejection, thus relieving symptoms like dyspnea on exertion, chest pain, or light-headedness.

208. The answer is C. *(Braunwald, ed 11. pp 923–925. Mandel, ed 2. pp 187, 199.)* The rhythm strip shown below, and in the question, demonstrates normal sinus rhythm with two atrial premature contractions (beats numbered 5 and 9). P waves of atrial premature contractions appear earlier than expected and differ in morphology from the P waves of the sinus beats. They may be conducted to the ventricles resulting in relatively normal-appearing QRS complexes or, if they occur during the refractory period of the ventricles, they may be blocked. In this situation, premature P waves would differ in morphology from the P waves of the sinus beats and no QRS complex would follow the P wave. Atrial premature contractions may occur singly or may result in atrial flutter, atrial fibrillation, or atrial tachycardia.

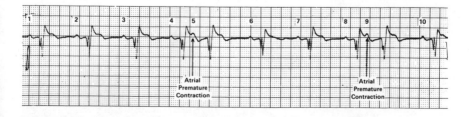

209. The answer is E. *(Braunwald, ed 11. pp 925–930. Mandel, ed 2. pp 224, 226, 228.)* Multifocal atrial tachycardia tends to occur in patients who have severe lung disease. It is characterized by varying P-wave morphology and P-R intervals. The rhythm strip shown below exhibits at least three different P-wave shapes. The beats numbered 8, 10, and 12 are probably aberrantly conducted, resulting in their more bizarre appearance. The presence of severe pulmonary disease in the patient from whom the strip was obtained is suggested by the tall, peaked P waves (P pulmonale).

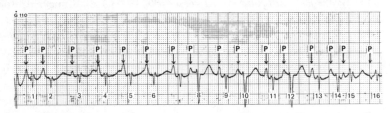

210. The answer is D. *(Braunwald, ed 11. pp 922, 926–938.)* In patients with atrial fibrillation, especially those with mitral stenosis, thromboembolic complications are common. Thromboembolism is responsible for about 20 percent of deaths in patients with mitral stenosis. Long-term anticoagulation therapy has been shown to be advantageous in the treatment of these patients. Anticoagulants should be given for at least 2 weeks before attempting to reinstate sinus rhythm. Sinus bradycardia is dangerous when ventricular premature beats are present; the low sinus rate facilitates the development of ventricular tachycardia. However, there is no agreement as to the best treatment of sinus bradycardia itself in patients who have experienced myocardial infarction. Indeed, some studies suggest that sinus bradycardia is indicative of a favorable prognosis. Ventricular tachycardia is a serious problem— lidocaine may be tried as the therapy of first choice if the dysrhythmia occurs soon after infarction and the patient has no undue distress. If 100 to 200 mg of intravenous lidocaine do not control the dysrhythmia, electrical conversion should be attempted. Quinidine, by enhancing atrioventricular conduction, may enhance ventricular rates in patients with atrial flutter. Thus, there is a need for digoxin or propranolol in quinidine-treated patients with atrial flutter.

211. The answer is A. *(Braunwald, ed 11. pp 643, 1038.)* Aneurysms of the aorta from syphilis occur most commonly in the ascending aorta and least commonly in the descending thoracic and abdominal aortae. Calcification in the wall of the ascending aorta is frequently present. Aneurysm formation occurs 15 to 30 years following infection with syphilis. Syphilis may affect the cardiovascular system in several additional ways. Aortic valvular insufficiency is the most common complication of syphilitic aortitis. In addition, syphilis may involve the coronary ostia resulting in progressive occlusion and symptoms of angina or myocardial infarction.

212. The answer is D. *(Braunwald, ed 11. pp 956–960. Hurst, ed 6. pp 754–764.)* The patient presented in the question has severe mitral stenosis as evidenced by her symptoms, physical examination, and calculated valve area of 0.8 cm² (normal range: 4 to 6 cm²). Because of her disabling symptoms, surgery should be recommended. A loud first heart sound and an opening snap imply a noncalcified, pliable mitral valve. These findings, together with the absence of mitral regurgitation, make this patient an ideal candidate for mitral valve commissurotomy. Commissurotomy is preferred to implantation of a prosthetic valve since the former procedure carries a lower risk and avoids the long-term complications of the anticoagulation therapy that valve replacement requires. Digitalis, in the absence of rapid atrial fibrillation, would not be of significant benefit. While anticoagulant therapy is not indicated in this patient at this time, the presence of intermittent atrial fibrillation or an embolic complication would mandate the use of an anticoagulant for at least 1 year.

213. The answer is C. *(Braunwald, ed 11. pp 993, 1011.)* Dressler's syndrome may develop following the escape of blood into the pericardial cavity from a variety of causes (e.g., cardiac surgery, myocardial infarction, trauma to the heart from a nonpenetrating blow to the chest, perforation of the heart by a pacemaking catheter). The syndrome usually occurs 2 to 4 weeks following the cardiac injury but quite frequently appears after a lapse of months, even years. Relapses are very common. Symptoms of Dressler's syndrome include fever, pleuritis, pericarditis, pneumonitis, arthritis, and leukocytosis. The syndrome, which is thought to be a result of immunological sensitization to cardiac antigens presented to lymphocytes at the time of the injury, correlates with the presence of antimyocardial antibodies; the clinical picture associated with the syndrome resembles that seen with both viral and idiopathic pericarditis. In the patient presented in the question, the history of a knife wound helps to eliminate those entities as diagnostic possibilities. Often no treatment other than mild analgesics is needed, but the problem can be very serious and even fatal. Severe cases usually respond to corticosteroids. Rheumatoid arthritis can be precipitated by trauma to joints and may be associated at the time of onset with an infection that appears to be viral. The age and sex of this particular patient makes a diagnosis of rheumatoid arthritis unlikely. While pleural effusions are relatively common in rheumatoid arthritis, pericardial effusions are rare. Bacterial endocarditis would be associated with all the patient's symptoms but clear evidence of endocardial disease would be required to support such a diagnosis.

214. The answer is B. *(Braunwald, ed 11. pp 963–966. Hurst, ed 6. pp 635–642.)* The patient discussed in the question has physical findings compatible with severe aortic stenosis. He probably has a congenital bicuspid valve that has progressively calcified. His heart signs suggest severe obstruction across the aortic valve. The fourth heart sound most likely results from contraction of the atrium against a thick, noncompliant left ventricle. Congestive failure, syncope, and chest pain indicate severe aortic stenosis; angina associated with aortic stenosis probably results from a thick, ischemic, left ventricular wall. Coronary artery disease coexisting with the aortic stenosis is an additional possibility. Cardiac catheterization is indicated to define the severity of the patient's aortic stenosis. Propranolol should not be used for this patient since the decrease in contractility produced by the drug may further reduce blood flow across the aortic valve.

215. The answer is B. *(Braunwald, ed 11. pp 977–979.)* Exercise testing under carefully controlled conditions can safely place a hemodynamic load on the myocardium that, in the presence of ischemic disease, will produce characteristic electrocardiographic changes. Because of the ability of stress testing to provide early warning of potential ischemic episodes in asymptomatic patients, its use in routine physical examinations, particularly in men over the age of 35, is rapidly increasing. Longitudinal studies of young personnel in the armed forces who had an abnormal exercise tolerance test, in spite of an absence of symptoms, have revealed that this group indeed is at risk for developing angina, myocardial infarction, and even sudden death. A diagnosis of ischemic heart disease by stress testing often can be followed by preventive measures that will delay or minimize subsequent clinical episodes of ischemic heart disease. The role of arteriography and corrective bypass surgery in such patients remains controversial and will not be settled until more data are available from longitudinal studies. In determining whether angiography is needed in a particular case, the following factors should be considered: (1) Were the abnormalities noted extreme? For example, a 4-mm ST-segment depression occurring after a short period of mild exercise is extreme. (2) In which electrocardiographic leads did the changes predominate? For example, changes in anterior leads have a worse prognosis than those in inferior leads. (3) What is the patient's age? (4) What is the patient's occupation? The pilot described in the question clearly should have angiography; a 75-year-old man, all things considered, probably should not.

216. The answer is D. *(Braunwald, ed 11. pp 972–975.)* In contrast to subacute bacterial endocarditis, acute bacterial endocarditis frequently develops on normal heart valves. While rheumatic and congenital malformations of the endocardium frequently act as predisposing factors for subacute bacterial endocarditis, general debilitation—especially that found in abusers of alcohol, drugs, or both—is more likely to be the predisposing factor in acute endocarditis. Acute bacterial endocarditis also is a risk for older men with chronic prostatitis, particularly at the time of surgery, or for women with genitourinary infections, particularly following abortion. Although endocardial destruction may be so severe and so rapid that emergency surgery is necessary, positive blood culture often will allow antibiotic therapy to be successfully introduced before surgery becomes necessary. In genitourinary infections, the invading organisms often are enterococci *(Streptococcus faecalis, S. faecium, S. durans)*. Because these microorganisms are relatively resistant to penicillin, a combination of penicillin and gentamicin, acting synergistically against enterococci, is recommended. A daily regimen of 12 to 24 million units of penicillin G and 3 to 5 mg/kg of gentamicin usually will suffice. When acute bacterial endocarditis is caused by group D nonenterococcal organisms such as *S. bovis,* penicillin alone is quite satisfactory. An additional advantage of penicillin is the avoidance of the potential toxic effects of gentamicin. In either situation, parenteral treatment must continue for a minimum of 4 weeks. In patients who are allergic to penicillin, vancomycin and streptomycin are usually successful.

217. The answer is C (2, 4). *(Braunwald, ed 11. pp 1012–1014.)* Constrictive pericarditis may follow almost any insult to the pericardium and is characterized by an obliteration of the pericardial cavity with consequent constriction of the heart and restriction of ventricular filling. Causes include trauma, infection, neoplasia, radiation, uremia, and connective tissue diseases; in many cases, no inciting event can be determined. The basic defect of this condition is an impairment of diastolic filling and a decrease in stroke volume; cardiac function may be normal. Patients typically present with fatigue, muscle wasting, and dyspnea on exertion; acute pulmonary edema is uncommon. Symptoms and signs of right-sided heart failure are present and include hepatomegaly, ascites, impaired lymphatic drainage from the small intestine leading to a protein-losing state, and dependent edema. A paradoxical pulse is found in one-third of patients and may be associated with Kussmaul's sign. The major problem in diagnosis is in differentiating constrictive pericarditis from the restrictive cardiomyopathies. In constrictive pericarditis, the left atrial pressure equals right atrial pressure, the cardiac output is only slightly depressed, and the right ventricular end diastolic pressure approaches one-third the systolic pressure. In the restrictive cardiomyopathies, left atrial pressure is greater than right atrial pressure, the cardiac output is usually significantly reduced, and the right ventricular end diastolic pressure is less than one-third the systolic pressure. Furthermore, echocardiography demonstrates pericardial thickening and paradoxical septal motion in patients with constrictive pericarditis. Treatment involves surgical resection of the pericardium; progressive improvement over several months commonly ensues.

218. The answer is B (1, 3). *(Hurst, ed 6. pp 1058–1059.)* Renovascular hypertension accounts for approximately 3 percent of the hypertensive population and the vast majority of cases are secondary to fibrous dysplasia or atherosclerosis of the renal artery. Fibrous dysplasia is most prevalent in women and is associated with an abdominal bruit in 60 percent of cases; in contrast, atherosclerotic renovascular disease occurs primarily in men over age 45. The onset of hypertension before age 30 or after age 50, the presence of grade 3 or 4 retinopathy, the sudden onset of severe hypertension, or the development of uncontrollable hypertension in a patient with previously controllable blood pressure all increase the likelihood of the hypertension's being renovascular. Once the presence of a lesion of the renal artery has been confirmed by either intravenous pyelogram, digital subtraction angiography, or renal arteriography, the functional significance of the stenosis is determined by measuring the renal vein renin ratio after sodium depletion. If the renal vein renin from the stenotic side exceeds the contralateral renal vein renin by 50 percent or more, then 90 percent of patients will have an improvement in blood pressure with surgical correction. This measurement, however, does not predict failure, as 50 percent of patients whose renins do not "lateralize" will also experience surgical improvement.

219. The answer is E (all). *(Hoshino, Arch Intern Med 146:349–352, 1986.)* Chronic aortic regurgitation generally progresses in slow fashion with very low mortality during a long asymptomatic phase; indeed, as many as 85 to 95 percent of patients with mild-to-moderate aortic insufficiency will survive for 10 years. This period of compensation is characterized by dilation of the left ventricular chamber, an increase in myocardial mass, and normal myocardial contractility. Once symptoms develop, however, there is rapid deterioration characterized by gross left ventricular enlargement with inadequate hypertrophy, high wall stress, and depressed myocardial contractility. Patients who develop congestive heart failure often expire within 2 years after onset of symptoms, while those with angina pectoris have an average survival of 5 years. Furthermore, a preoperative ejection fraction of 45 percent and a cardiac index above 2.5 L/min/m² are associated with a higher postoperative survival than an ejection fraction less than 45 percent and a cardiac index less than 2.5 L/min/m². Because prognosis is related to ventricular function, recommendations for aortic valve replacement can be made. Symptomatic patients, and asymptomatic patients with evidence of left ventricular dysfunction at rest as measured by radionuclide studies or echocardiography, should have surgery. Asymptomatic patients who demonstrate left ventricular dysfunction only with exercise should probably have surgery as well. The early mortality for aortic valve replacement for patients with aortic regurgitation is approximately 2 to 3 percent.

220. The answer is B (1, 3). *(Rackley, pp 181–191.)* Cardiac tamponade is characterized by a sufficient rise in intrapericardial pressure to cause a decrease in cardiac filling, a reduced cardiac output, and peripheral hypoperfusion. Causes include trauma, malignancy (most commonly lung and breast cancers), infection, uremia, connective tissue diseases, and radiation therapy. Patients present with symptoms of visceral and hepatic congestion, dyspnea, and chest discomfort. On examination, tachycardia, an elevated jugular venous pressure, a paradoxical pulse, and a narrow pulse pressure are seen; Kussmaul's sign is uncommon in cardiac tamponade. Diagnosis is best made by echocardiography. Treatment involves fluid expansion, vasodilation, and pericardiocentesis.

221–223. The answers are: 221-D, 222-B, 223-A. *(Braunwald, ed 11. pp 966–969, 1012–1014. Hurst, ed 6. pp 745–746, 795, 1263.)* Tricuspid stenosis is characterized by a slow *y* descent of the jugular pulse and a diastolic rumble at the lower left sternal border.

Aortic regurgitation, in addition to generating the characteristic decrescendo diastolic murmur along the left sternal border, may also cause a diastolic rumble at the apex. Termed an Austin Flint murmur, this diastolic rumble is thought to result from the regurgitant jet of blood hitting the anterior leaflet of the mitral valve. Although distinguishing this murmur from that of mitral stenosis may be difficult, the absence of both an opening snap and loud first heart sound should suggest an Austin Flint murmur.

Constrictive pericarditis is characterized by a sharp y descent; this diagnosis should be considered in any patient who has unexplained edema or ascites.

224–227. The answers are: 224-D, 225-C, 226-A, 227-B. *(Braunwald, ed 11. pp 1031–1036.)* Drugs used in the treatment of hypertension fall into four distinct classes: diuretics, antiadrenergic agents, vasodilators, and angiotensin blockers. Captopril, by inhibiting the angiotensin converting enzyme, is a potent antihypertensive agent because it prevents the generation of angiotensin II, a vasoconstrictor, and inhibits the degradation of bradykinin, a vasodilator. While especially useful in renovascular hypertension, it may cause membranous glomerulopathy, the nephrotic syndrome, and leukopenia.

Hydralazine is an arterial vasodilator generally used in conjunction with drugs that prevent reflex sympathetic stimulation of the heart, such as beta blockers and methyldopa. A lupuslike syndrome has been produced with doses exceeding 300 mg per day.

Propranolol is a nonselective beta blocker and may therefore cause bronchospasm in susceptible patients. Beta blockers, as a class, may reduce HDL cholesterol and increase serum triglyceride levels.

Minoxidil is a more potent vasodilator than hydralazine but its use is limited by the high incidence of hirsutism. Marked fluid retention also occurs.

Gynecomastia is not a side effect of the drugs listed, although spironolactone, a potassium-sparing diuretic, and methyldopa, a centrally acting antiadrenergic agent, are two antihypertensives that may cause this side effect.

228–231. The answers are: 228-E, 229-D, 230-B, 231-A. *(Braunwald, ed 11. pp 880–881. Hurst, ed 6. pp 1466–1477.)* Hypokalemia typically increases automaticity of myocardial fibers, resulting in ectopic beats or arrhythmias. Electrocardiography in hypokalemia reveals flattening of the T wave and prominent U waves.

Hyperkalemia decreases the rate of spontaneous diastolic depolarization in all pacemaker cells. It also results in slowing of conduction. One of the earliest electrocardiographic signs of hyperkalemia is the appearance of tall, peaked T waves. More severe elevations of the serum potassium result in widening of the QRS complex.

Hypocalcemia results in prolongation of the Q-T interval, most commonly when the serum calcium level falls below 6 mg/100 ml. Low serum calcium levels tend to decrease myocardial contractility.

At serum sodium levels compatible with life, neither hyponatremia nor hypernatremia results in any characteristic electrocardiographic abnormalities.

232–236. The answers are: 232-A, 233-D, 234-E, 235-B, 236-A. *(Braunwald, ed 11. pp 866–867. Hurst, ed 6. pp 147–150.)* The normal jugular venous pulse wave consists of three positive waves and two troughs. Normally, the *a* wave is the largest wave and is due to right atrial contraction. The *c* wave that follows is probably related to bulging of the tricuspid valve into the atrium. Relaxation of the atrium results in the *x* descent. The *v* wave results from the filling of the right atrium with blood while the tricuspid valve is still closed. The *y* descent is the result of opening of the tricuspid valve. An S_4 gallop is produced by atrial contraction and thus would occur at approximately the same time as the *a* wave.

Thus, abnormally large *a* waves would be expected in situations in which the right atrium is contracting against increased resistance such as tricuspid stenosis, pulmonic stenosis, or pulmonary hypertension. Moderate or severe tricuspid regurgitation typically causes obliteration of the normal *x* descent. When regurgitation is severe, the *c* and *v* waves may merge, resulting in a single, large *v* wave. Obstruction to right atrial emptying would be expected to result in a slow *y* descent, which is classically seen with tricuspid stenosis. A prominent *y* descent is characteristic of constrictive pericarditis.

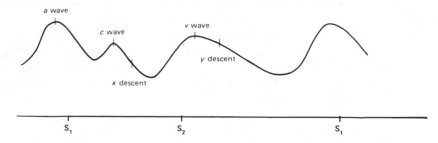

237–239. The answers are: 237-A, 238-D, 239-C. *(Braunwald, ed 11. pp 940, 1611–1614, 2034.)* Dextrocardia is a prominent feature of Kartagener's syndrome, an inherited condition that features situs inversus, chronic sinusitis, and bronchiectasis.

Aortic and pulmonary artery dilatation commonly occur with homocystinuria, an inborn error of metabolism. This condition, which is caused by a deficiency of the enzyme cystathionine synthetase, is characterized by the presence of intravascular thrombosis, lens subluxation, and osteoporosis, as well as large-vessel dilatation.

Hyperextensible joints, one of the common defects in Down's syndrome (trisomy 21), are frequently associated with cardiac abnormalities, including an endocardial cushion defect, atrial and ventricular septal defects, and the tetralogy of Fallot. Hypotonia often accompanies the hyperextensible joints. Mongoloid facies and mental retardation are regularly associated with this syndrome.

Endocrinology and Metabolic Disease

DIRECTIONS: Each question below contains five suggested responses. Select the **one best** response to each question.

240. A 15-½-year-old boy and his parents are concerned about the absence of any signs of puberty. His friends have all entered puberty and he feels embarrassed. He is nervous but well and his growth curves for height and weight are adequate. The physician asks the boy if his ability to smell is impaired. He thinks it is but as he did not volunteer the information his physician is uncertain of the significance of the answer. Physical examination is unrevealing. His physician should now recommend that

(A) urine and plasma levels of follicle-stimulating hormone (FSH) and luteinizing hormone (LH) be obtained
(B) the boy come back in a year for a further evaluation, as delayed puberty in boys is so common that it would be premature to investigate the matter further
(C) cortisol, testosterone, and thyroid hormone levels be measured and an x-ray of the sella turcica be obtained
(D) a gonadorelin stimulation test be performed to rule out a deficiency of luteinizing releasing hormone (LRH)
(E) a skeletal survey be done to look for the classic radiological clues to Kallmann's syndrome

241. A 42-year-old woman is evaluated for hypoglycemia. She has experienced recurrent episodes of inappropriate behavior and dizziness for the past year, and she had syncope on one occasion after mowing her lawn. She denies hunger or palpitations and only occasionally has noted sweating. The patient has gained 15 pounds during the last year. Laboratory plasma studies reveal a glucose level of 65 mg/100 ml, insulin level of 18 μU/ml (normal: 10 to 20) after an overnight fast, and a diabetic glucose tolerance test (2-hour value: 225 mg/100 ml) without reactive hypoglycemia. After 48 hours of fasting, the patient became confused. At this time her plasma glucose and insulin levels are 34 mg/100 ml and 20 μU/ml, respectively. The most likely diagnosis is

(A) Addison's disease
(B) reactive hypoglycemia
(C) diabetes mellitus
(D) insulinoma
(E) hepatoma

242. The patient pictured below complains of the sudden onset of a painful "lump" in her neck following an upper respiratory infection. Physical examination reveals a soft, round, tender, midline mass at the level of the hyoid bone. The most likely diagnosis is

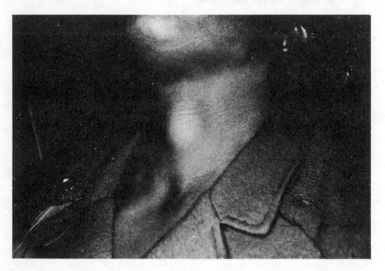

(A) acute suppurative thyroiditis
(B) subacute thyroiditis
(C) thyroglossal duct cyst
(D) toxic nodular goiter
(E) thyroid adenoma

243. It is estimated that 50 million women use oral contraceptives; however, concerns about short- and long-term toxicity remain a major problem. A physician is presenting to a patient contemplating the use of an oral contraceptive current knowledge of the potential side effects she may encounter. All the following statements are accurate EXCEPT that

(A) nausea is common at the beginning of therapy but usually ceases to be a problem after the second cycle of pills

(B) the risk of developing ovarian and endometrial cancer may be reduced by as much as 50 percent by using oral contraceptive preparations that contain both estrogen and progestin

(C) long-term follow-up studies that have now reached 20 years have found that there is no increase in the incidence of breast cancer in women taking oral contraceptives and that indeed benign breast lesions occur less frequently

(D) oral contraceptives should be stopped 1 month before elective surgery

(E) with the lowering of the estrogen content in combination preparations the incidence of venous thromboses has been reduced. Long-term studies have confirmed initial suspicions that combination preparations are associated with arterial thromboses

244. A 25-year-old woman who has insulin-dependent diabetes develops recurrent hypoglycemia. Her history reveals amenorrhea of 2 months' duration. A urinalysis is negative for glucose and protein; a vaginal smear shows no evidence of estrogen deficiency. The most likely diagnosis is

(A) pregnancy
(B) renal failure
(C) hypopituitarism
(D) insulinoma
(E) hyperthyroidism

245. A 30-year-old man is evaluated for a thyroid nodule. The patient reports that his father died from "thyroid cancer" and that a brother had a history of recurrent renal stones. Blood calcitonin concentration is 2000 pg/ml (normal: less than 100); serum calcium and phosphate levels are normal. Before referring the patient to a surgeon, the physician should

(A) obtain a liver scan
(B) perform a calcium infusion test
(C) measure urinary catecholamines
(D) administer suppressive doses of thyroxine and measure levels of thyroid stimulating hormone
(E) treat the patient with radioactive iodine

246. A 27-year-old woman presents with shortness of breath. Her radiological skeletal survey is negative. Laboratory serum values are as follows:

> Chloride: 98 mEq/L
> Calcium: 11.9 mg/100 ml (normal: 9 to 11)
> Phosphorus: 3.6 mg/100 ml (normal: 3 to 4.5)
> Uric acid: 8.5 mg/100 ml (normal 1.5 to 6.0)
> Alkaline phosphatase: 50 U/L (normal 21–91)

Blood urea nitrogen is 20 mg/100 ml. Pulmonary function tests reveal reduced vital capacity and reduced carbon monoxide diffusing capacity. Flat plate x-ray of the abdomen reveals bilateral nephrocalcinosis. The appropriate treatment for this patient is

(A) parathyroid exploration followed by subtotal parathyroidectomy
(B) potassium phosphate, 2 g daily
(C) mithramycin, 25 µg/kg body weight
(D) cyclophosphamide, 2 mg/kg daily
(E) prednisone, 50 mg daily

247. A patient develops severe hypotension immediately after removal of a pheochromocytoma. The most appropriate management would be the administration of which of the following?

(A) Corticosteroids
(B) Mineralocorticoids
(C) Alpha-stimulating agents
(D) Beta-stimulating agents
(E) Blood or plasma

248. A 25-year-old woman with a history of normal onset of menses is found on physical examination to have a blood pressure of 175/110, clitoromegaly, and hirsutism. Laboratory values reveal a potassium of 3.0 and depressed aldosterone and plasma renin activity levels. The likely diagnosis for this patient is

(A) 11 β-hydroxylase deficiency
(B) 17 α-hydroxylase deficiency
(C) Addison's disease
(D) 21-hydroxylase deficiency
(E) none of the above

249. An otherwise healthy 60-year-old man is noted on routine examination to have a firm thyroid nodule. Serum thyroxine is 8.0 µg/100 ml (normal: 4 to 11). Thyroid scan demonstrates a "cold" nodule, and ultrasonography reveals that the mass is solid. The most appropriate management would be which of the following procedures?

(A) Complete lobectomy
(B) Needle biopsy
(C) Exogenous thyroid suppression
(D) Radioactive iodine therapy
(E) External irradiation

250. A 54-year-old man who has had a Billroth II procedure for peptic ulcer disease now presents with abdominal pain and is found to have recurrent ulcer disease. The physician is considering this patient's illness to be secondary either to a retained antrum or to a gastrinoma. Which of the following tests would best differentiate the two conditions?

(A) Random gastrin level
(B) 24-Hour acid production determination
(C) Serum calcium level
(D) Secretin infusion
(E) Insulin-induced hypoglycemia

251. A 60-year-old woman who has been aware of a swelling in her neck for many years presents with generalized muscle weakness, loss of appetite, and palpitations. An electrocardiogram reveals rapid atrial fibrillation. Despite adequate digitalization, there is little slowing of her ventricular rate. Thyroid function studies reveal a serum thyroxine level of 12 μg/100 ml (normal: 5 to 12), with a triiodothyronine (T_3) level of 200 ng/100 ml (normal: 80 to 160), as measured by radioimmunoassay. In respect to this patient's disorder, the most appropriate diagnosis and treatment would be

(A) typical Graves' disease; therapy with antithyroid drugs
(B) toxic multinodular goiter; therapy with antithyroid drugs followed by surgery
(C) toxic multinodular goiter; initiation of therapy with 10 μCi/g of ^{131}I
(D) toxic multinodular goiter; initiation of therapy with antithyroid agents followed by 20 μCi/g of ^{131}I when euthyroid
(E) toxic multinodular goiter; initiation of therapy with propranolol and antithyroid agents followed by 20 μCi of ^{131}I when euthyroid

252. A 35-year-old woman has a 6-month history of amenorrhea. A 5-day course of medroxyprogesterone acetate (Provera), 10 mg, fails to induce withdrawal bleeding, while vaginal bleeding occurs following 20 days of conjugated estrogen (1.25 mg) administration. Her serum luteinizing and follicle-stimulating hormones are markedly increased. These findings are most consistent with which of the following abnormalities?

(A) Pituitary adenoma
(B) Polycystic ovary syndrome
(C) Endometrial failure
(D) Premature menopause
(E) Psychiatric illness

253. A 32-year-old woman has a 3-year history of oligomenorrhea that has progressed to amenorrhea during the past year. She has observed loss of breast fullness, reduced hip measurements, acne, increased body hair, and deepening of her voice. Physical examination reveals frontal balding, clitoral hypertrophy, and a male escutcheon. Urinary 17-hydroxycorticoid and 17-ketosteroid levels are normal. Her plasma testosterone level is 6 ng/ml (normal: 0.2 to 0.8). The most likely diagnosis of this patient's disorder is

(A) hilar cell tumor
(B) Cushing's syndrome
(C) arrhenoblastoma
(D) polycystic ovary syndrome
(E) granulosa-theca cell tumor

254. A 55-year-old woman who has a history of severe depression and who had radical mastectomy for carcinoma of the breast 1 year previously develops polyuria, nocturia, and excessive thirst. Laboratory values are as follow:

Serum electrolytes (mEq/L):
  Na^+ 149; K^+ 3.6
Serum calcium: 9.5 mg/100 ml
Blood glucose: 110 mg/100 ml
Blood urea nitrogen: 30 mg/100 ml
Urine osmolality: 150 mOsm/kg

The most likely diagnosis is

(A) psychogenic polydipsia
(B) renal glycosuria
(C) hypercalciuria
(D) diabetes insipidus
(E) inappropriate antidiuretic hormone syndrome

255. An active 24-year-old woman is found to have Hodgkin's disease on the basis of a cervical node biopsy. Chest x-ray reveals an anterior mediastinal mass, but lymphangiogram and liver biopsy are negative. Radiotherapy to the involved lymph nodes results in clinical remission; however, 2 months later the patient develops clinical and laboratory evidence of hypothyroidism. The most likely cause for hypothyroidism in this patient is

(A) Hashimoto's thyroiditis
(B) iodine deficiency
(C) iodine excess
(D) lymphomatous infiltration of the thyroid
(E) hypopituitarism

DIRECTIONS: Each question below contains four suggested responses of which **one or more** is correct. Select

A	if	**1, 2, and 3**	are correct
B	if	**1 and 3**	are correct
C	if	**2 and 4**	are correct
D	if	**4**	is correct
E	if	**1, 2, 3, and 4**	are correct

256. A 45-year-old man is noted on physical examination to have coarse facial features, oily skin, and an enlarged tongue. Initial laboratory studies reveal a fasting glucose of 190 mg/100 ml. Which of the following would support the physician's presumptive diagnosis of acromegaly?

(1) An increase in growth hormone with oral glucose administration

(2) An increase in growth hormone with thyrotropin releasing hormone (TRH) administration

(3) Suppression of growth hormone with L-dopa administration

(4) A large sleep-related peak in growth hormone secretion

257. Correct statements concerning Turner's syndrome include which of the following?

(1) One in 2500 newborn females has gonadal dysgenesis

(2) Ten to twenty percent of victims of gonadal dysgenesis have a coarctation of the aorta

(3) Primitive gonads should be removed to avoid the risk of malignancy in patients who have Y chromosomal elements

(4) Early therapy with growth hormone will allow patients to avoid the short stature (150 cm or less) that is a feature of the natural disease

258. A thin, 30-year-old woman complains of nervousness, mild sweating, palpitations, scanty menses, and weight loss. Her blood pressure is 150/80 mm Hg and pulse rate 96/minute. She displays mild hyperpigmentation and telangiectasis on the face. A small thyroid nodule is palpable. Serum thyroxine is 9.0 μg/100 ml (normal: 4.5 to 10); resin T_3 uptake is normal; radioactive iodine uptake is 30 percent (normal: 5 to 35); and thyroid scan shows uptake by a solitary left-sided thyroid nodule (no uptake by the right lobe). The diagnosis of hyperthyroidism in this patient may be established by

(1) T_3 suppression test

(2) serum long-acting thyroid stimulator assay

(3) serum triiodothyronine radioimmunoassay

(4) serum thyroid-stimulating hormone assay

SUMMARY OF DIRECTIONS

A	B	C	D	E
1,2,3	1,3	2,4	4	All are
only	only	only	only	correct

259. Correct statements concerning the management of thyroid storm include that

(1) despite proper management, mortality is 20 percent
(2) saturated solution of potassium iodide (SSKI) immediately retards the release of thyroid hormones
(3) dexamethasone inhibits the generation of T_3 from T_4
(4) methimazole is as efficacious as propylthiouracil

260. Correct statements regarding the laboratory findings in patients who have Cushing's syndrome include which of the following?

(1) The presence of an abnormal diurnal steroid rhythm is diagnostic of the disorder
(2) An abnormal overnight dexamethasone suppression test (1 mg) is diagnostic of the disorder
(3) An exaggerated increase in plasma cortisol is usually observed following insulin-induced hypoglycemia
(4) Normal urinary 17-hydroxycorticosteroids are observed in 10 to 15 percent of affected patients

261. A 20-year-old man who has a history of polyuria and hypotonic urine is placed on restricted water intake. After a period of dehydration his urine osmolality stabilizes at 450 mOsm/kg. Following injection of vasopressin (Pitressin) his urine osmolality rises to 600 mOsm/kg. This patient's symptoms are likely to improve if he is treated with

(1) oral chlorpropamide
(2) thiazide diuretics
(3) lysine-vasopressin nasal spray
(4) oral tolbutamide

262. Correct statements about male infertility include which of the following?

(1) It can be associated with repeated respiratory tract infections
(2) The measurement of urinary 17-ketosteroids is a valuable way to assess the adequacy of testosterone production
(3) A low plasma testosterone level necessitates a repeat measurement with simultaneous assessment of luteinizing hormone
(4) Plasma follicle-stimulating hormone levels are useful, as the concentration of this hormone correlates directly with spermatogenesis

263. A patient who has undergone bilateral adrenalectomy for Cushing's syndrome develops a deep tan in winter. In evaluating this patient, the physician should consider the possibility of

(1) residual ectopic adrenal tissue
(2) a pituitary tumor
(3) iatrogenic Cushing's syndrome
(4) inadequate adrenal replacement

264. Hyperparathyroidism is associated with which of the following abnormalities?

(1) Moniliasis
(2) Personality disturbances
(3) Prolonged Q-T interval on electrocardiogram
(4) Intense pruritus

265. Gynecomastia is associated with which of the following situations?

(1) Cirrhosis
(2) Digitalis administration
(3) Puberty
(4) Hyperthyroidism

266. A 42-year-old man complains of impotence. His physician discovers that he is taking a drug that is known to interfere with the hormonal control of erection. Drugs having such an effect include

(1) chlorpheniramine
(2) spironolactone
(3) azathioprine
(4) cimetidine

267. A 25-year-old woman complains of a recent onset of nervousness, palpitations, and increased sweating. Her serum thyroxine is 15 μg/100 ml (normal: 4 to 11), and radioactive iodine uptake is 1 percent. Hyperthyroidism in this patient may have been induced by

(1) exogenous thyroid
(2) pituitary adenoma
(3) cholecystography
(4) oat-cell carcinoma of the lungs

268. A 30-year-old man complains of headaches. A skull x-ray shows enlargement of the sella turcica. These findings are consistent with a diagnosis of

(1) pituitary adenoma
(2) craniopharyngioma
(3) empty-sella syndrome
(4) internal carotid artery aneurysm

269. After an initial 2 to 3 hours of insulin treatment for diabetic ketoacidosis, there is most often a significant decline in blood level of

(1) glucose
(2) β-hydroxybutyrate
(3) free fatty acids
(4) acetoacetate

270. Cushing's syndrome is characterized by which of the following statements?

(1) Circulating eosinophils are below 100 cells/mm^3 in 90 percent of cases
(2) Although truncal obesity is generally present, a redistribution of weight is characteristic and approximately half the affected patients exhibit no weight gain
(3) Adrenal hyperplasia secondary to either pituitary or nonendocrine ACTH production can often be distinguished by a high-dosage dexamethasone suppression test
(4) The dexamethasone suppression test is less useful in screening for this syndrome than the now generally available radioimmunoassay for ACTH

271. Correct statements concerning diabetic retinopathy include which of the following?

(1) Cotton wool exudates represent microinfarcts
(2) Hard exudates reflect old, healed microinfarcts
(3) A sudden increase in the number of cotton wool exudates is a serious prognostic sign
(4) Cotton wool exudates are much more common than hard exudates

272. Hyperaldosteronism is often associated with

(1) diuretic therapy
(2) Cushing's syndrome
(3) malignant hypertension
(4) licorice ingestion

273. Hypercalcemia in sarcoidosis is associated with

(1) seasonal changes in serum calcium
(2) improvement following corticosteroid therapy
(3) reduced parathormone concentration
(4) brown tumors

274. X-ray findings associated with hyperparathyroidism include

(1) subperiosteal resorption of the phalanges
(2) pseudofractures
(3) dissolution of phalangeal tufts
(4) osteosclerosis

275. Toxic nodular goiter (Plummer's disease) is associated with

(1) exophthalmos
(2) thyroid acropathy
(3) pretibial myxedema
(4) onycholysis

276. A 26-year-old mother of one child, born 2 years ago, complains to her physician that she is embarrassed by the fact that sexual excitement is always associated with the leakage of milk from her nipples. She breast fed her baby for only 3 months. In discussing the evaluation and treatment of this problem with medical students, the physician would be correct in reporting that

(1) many cases are associated with increased levels of circulating prolactin, but that alone will not cause galactorrhea unless the woman has been previously primed by a pregnancy
(2) troublesome cases can frequently be controlled with the drug bromocriptine mesylate
(3) the finding of hyperprolactinemia is an indication that a work-up for a possible pituitary tumor is mandatory
(4) alpha methyldopa may interfere with the action of prolactin inhibitory hormone, thus facilitating galactorrhea

277. A 15-year-old boy, hospitalized for a fractured pelvis, is restricted to complete bedrest. Which of the following laboratory abnormalities may result?

(1) Glucose intolerance
(2) Hypercalcemia
(3) Absent diurnal steroid rhythm
(4) Hyperparathyroidism

278. Correct statements concerning diabetes insipidus include which of the following?

(1) A dehydration test requires withholding fluids until there is a loss in body weight of at least 4 kg
(2) Desmopressin acetate (DDAVP) is more effective than synthetic lypressin (DIAPID) in that its effect lasts from 12 to 24 hours
(3) Ethacrynic acid provides effective therapy
(4) Water intoxication with normal diluting capacity has been reported in patients given thioridazine (Mellaril)

279. Correct statements about thyroid antibodies include which of the following?

(1) They may be observed in 20 percent of elderly women
(2) They may be observed in 50 percent of patients with pernicious anemia
(3) They are usually observed in Hashimoto's thyroiditis
(4) They are usually observed in subacute thyroiditis

280. Correct statements concerning subacute thyroiditis (de Quervain's thyroiditis) include which of the following?

(1) Pain, both localized and referred, is characteristic
(2) The erythrocyte sedimentation rate is increased and radioactive iodine uptake decreased
(3) The thyroid is extremely tender and occasionally nodular
(4) An elevated protein-bound iodine level is commonly found

281. Active patients afflicted with Paget's disease (osteitis deformans) generally demonstrate elevated levels of which of the following substances?

(1) Serum alkaline phosphatase
(2) Serum calcium
(3) Urine hydroxyproline
(4) Urine calcium

DIRECTIONS: Each group of questions below consists of lettered headings followed by a set of numbered items. For each numbered item select the **one** lettered heading with which it is **most** closely associated. Each lettered heading may be used **once, more than once, or not at all.**

Questions 282–285

For each case presentation below, select the most appropriate diagnosis. (Laboratory values appear in the table below.)

(A) Adrenal carcinoma
(B) Congenital adrenal hyperplasia
(C) Cushing's syndrome
(D) Oat-cell carcinoma of the lung
(E) Nelson's syndrome

282. A 45-year-old man complains of severe weakness. He appears chronically wasted and is mildly hyperpigmented. His blood pressure is 160/100 mm Hg. A high-dose dexamethasone suppression test (2 mg every 6 hours) causes no suppression of urinary 17-hydroxycorticosteroids (17-OHCS) or 17-ketosteroids (17-KS)

283. A 26-year-old woman complains of irregular menses, obesity, and low back pain. She has mild hypertension, central obesity, broad striae, acne, and mild hirsutism. A low-dose dexamethasone suppression test (0.5 mg every 6 hours) causes no suppression of urinary 17-OHCS. A high-dose dexamethasone suppression test causes greater than 50 percent suppression of urinary 17-OHCS

284. A 20-year-old woman complains of weakness, easy bruising, hirsutism, and irregular menses. She exhibits a moon face, central obesity, and severe hirsutism involving the face and trunk, but no virilism. A high-dose dexamethasone suppression test causes no suppression of 17-OHCS or 17-KS

285. A 15-year-old boy complains of short stature. He has a history of early sexual development and accelerated growth that ceased 5 years ago. He displays hyperpigmentation. A high-dose dexamethasone suppression test causes greater than 50 percent suppression of urinary 17-KS

Laboratory Values

Patient Number	Serum K+ (mEq/L)	Serum HCO₃ (mEq/L)	Plasma Cortisol at 6 P.M. (µg/100 ml)*	Plasma ACTH (pg/100 ml)†	Urine 17-OHCS (mg/24 hr)★	Urine 17-KS (mg/24 hr)‡
282.	3.0	35	40	1000	35	40
283.	3.9	25	20	90	15	15
284.	3.2	32	80	5	35	70
285.	3.8	25	13	250	4	65

*Normal: 10 to 24.
†Normal: 40 to 100.
★Normal: 3 to 12.
‡Normal: male < 20; female < 1.5.

Questions 286–289

For each case presentation below, select the lipoprotein disorder with which it is most closely associated.

(A) Hyperchylomicronemia (type I)
(B) Hyperbetalipoproteinemia (type IIa)
(C) "Broad-beta" disease (type III)
(D) Hyperprebetalipoproteinemia (type IV)
(E) Combined hyperlipoproteinemia (type IIb)

286. A 45-year-old diabetic patient complains of intermittent claudication. Physical examination reveals xanthomas of the palmar and digital creases and tuberoeruptive xanthomas of the elbows. Serum cholesterol and triglycerides are 320 and 280 mg/100 ml, respectively

287. A 12-year-old girl complains of acute abdominal pain. Physical examination reveals eruptive xanthomas, hepatosplenomegaly, and lipemia retinalis. Blood drawn on hospital admission looks like "cream of tomato soup"

288. A 32-year-old man has chest pain on exertion and a strong family history of coronary artery disease. Xanthomas are present on his Achilles tendon. Serum cholesterol and triglycerides are 380 and 150 mg/100 ml, respectively

289. A 24-year-old woman is treated with oral contraceptives. Routine blood studies reveal turbid plasma

DIRECTIONS: Each group of questions below consists of four lettered headings followed by a set of numbered items. For each numbered item select

A	if the item is associated with	(A) **only**
B	if the item is associated with	(B) **only**
C	if the item is associated with	**both** (A) and (B)
D	if the item is associated with	**neither** (A) nor (B)

Each lettered heading may be used **once, more than once, or not at all.**

Questions 290–294

(A) Multiple endocrine neoplasia, type I (MEN I)
(B) Multiple endocrine neoplasia, type II (MEN II)
(C) Both
(D) Neither

290. Medullary thyroid carcinoma

291. Multicentric parathyroid involvement

292. Increased ratio of urinary epinephrine to norepinephrine

293. Peptic ulcer disease is the major cause of morbidity and mortality

294. Carcinoid tumors

Questions 295–299

(A) Propylthiouracil (PTU)
(B) Methimazole
(C) Both
(D) Neither

295. Decrease in the peripheral conversion of T_4 to T_3

296. Inhibition of the incorporation of iodide into thyroglobulin

297. Leukopenia

298. Interference with the release of previously formed thyroid hormone

299. Intrathyroidal concentrations reflected by serum levels

Endocrinology and Metabolic Disease

Answers

240. The answer is D. *(Braunwald, ed 11. pp 1811–1813. Med Lett Drugs Ther 25:106, 1983.)* A delay in the onset of puberty is much more common in boys than in girls and is usually a psychological hazard that can be handled with appropriate counseling. Genetic factors are important, and a history of delayed puberty in a father or an older brother would strongly suggest that no further investigations are needed. A physician would obviously look for signs of malnutrition from primary or secondary causes, as this can certainly affect the onset of puberty. It is important, however, to diagnose and treat as early as possible idiopathic gonadotropin deficiency. This problem can arise if there is a lack of the normal secretion by the hypothalamus of luteinizing hormone release factor (LHRF). Such a defect can occur in association with other symptoms and signs such as anosmia and skeletal deformities that cluster together as Kallmann's syndrome. Recently, a synthetic luteinizing releasing hormone, gonadorelin, has been approved by the FDA for diagnostic assessment of such cases. After the administration of this synthetic hormone, levels of FSH and LH are measured. Higher levels of these hormones after the administration of the LHRF strongly suggest the deficiency of the naturally occurring hormone. Midline facial deformities may occur in Kallmann's syndrome, and skeletal anomalies have been reported in a few cases. A radiological survey of the skeleton is not necessary, however; when delayed puberty in boys is caused by pituitary disease, a tumor on or above the sella turcica is the most likely cause. Visual defects such as bitemporal hemianopia are common. As pituitary disorders are usually acquired rather than congenital, the effects tend to be seen at a later stage in life. Impotence is usually the first endocrine manifestation in most adult males that pituitary insufficiency may be present. The absence of growth hormone usually does not produce significant symptoms in young adults.

241. The answer is D. *(Braunwald, ed 11. p 1382. Felig, ed 2. pp 1184–1187.)* The case history presented in the question is classic for insulinoma. The predominance of exercise-induced hypoglycemia and weight gain is characteristic of this disorder. Affected patients may have plasma insulin levels within normal limits after an overnight fast and frequently have glucose intolerance after glucose ingestion. The failure of insulin to fall when fasting hypoglycemia develops establishes the diagnosis of hyperinsulinism. In contrast, patients having reactive hypoglycemia do not develop hypoglycemia with fasting. Although hepatoma and Addison's disease may be associated with fasting hypoglycemia, insulin values fall appropriately during a fast in these disorders.

242. The answer is C. *(Braunwald, ed 11. pp 1732–1733.)* Thyroglossal duct cyst is the most important anomaly of thyroid development. Excision of the cyst is generally indicated because of the cyst's propensity for infection. Infection may enter the duct if a communication persists with the pharynx through the foramen cecum at the base of the tongue. After an acute upper respiratory infection, the duct may become obstructed. The obstruction can lead to cystic dilatation, thereby making the lesion clinically apparent.

243. The answer is E. *(Braunwald, ed 11. pp 1832–1834.)* Considering the extraordinarily large number of women using oral contraceptives it is surprising that it has taken so long to learn more about the risks associated with the use of these preparations. The high-dose sequential tablets have been removed from the market as clear evidence revealed that their use caused an increase in endometrial cancer. There is no evidence that the combined oral contraceptive preparations containing estrogen and progestin are associated with an increased incidence of cancer. Oral contraceptives would be contraindicated in a patient who has a malignancy that is sensitive to these hormones. The major risks associated with the use of modern oral contraceptive preparations continue to be vascular ones. It is true that as the estrogen content has progressively been reduced to the minimum level that will suppress gonadotropin secretion and yet prevent breakthrough bleeding, the incidence of venous thromboses has decreased. The use of these preparations, however, is still associated with a four-to-tenfold increase in the risk of developing a thrombosis. Previous evidence of thrombotic disease, obesity, heart failure, or immobilization will significantly increase the risk. Unfortunately, the incidence of arterial thrombosis does not appear to have improved with the lowering of the estrogen content in oral contraceptives. Oral contraceptives should be discontinued 1 month before elective surgery because their use is associated with increased risk of postoperative thromboembolism. Women over the age of 35 years who smoke cigarettes and use oral contraceptives definitely have an increased risk of myocardial infarction. In addition, thromboses are likely to occur in vessels that are rarely the site of symptomatic disease in young women, for example mesenteric and cerebral vessels. Even without the increased risk associated with smoking many physicians are now recommending that the use of oral contraceptives by women over the age of 35 should be discouraged. Absolute contraindications to the use of oral contraceptives include impaired liver function, pregnancy, undiagnosed vaginal bleeding, and hyperlipidemic states.

244. The answer is A. *(Braunwald, ed 11. p 1785. Felig, ed 2. pp 1155–1162.)* During the first trimester of pregnancy, diabetic women are particularly prone to hypoglycemia, a propensity that has been ascribed to fetal utilization of glucose and gluconeogenic substrates. Later in pregnancy, insulin requirements increase owing to a rise in placental contrainsular hormones. In the patient presented in the question, diabetic nephropathy is highly unlikely because of the absence of proteinuria. Owing to the lack of evidence of estrogen deficiency on vaginal smear, hypopituitarism also is unlikely.

245. The answer is C. *(Braunwald, ed 11. pp 1853–1854. Felig, ed 2. pp 1670–1675.)* For the patient described in the question, the markedly increased calcitonin levels indicate the diagnosis of medullary carcinoma of the thyroid. However, in view of the family history, the patient may also have a pheochromocytoma (multiple endocrine adenomatosis, type 2). These tumors sometimes are associated with an excess of catecholamines. Before thyroid surgery is performed on this patient, a pheochromocytoma must be ruled out through urinary catecholamine determinations; the presence of such a tumor might expose him to a hypertensive crisis during surgery. The entire thyroid gland must be removed, owing to the presence of numerous small and possibly malignant adenomata scattered throughout the gland. Successful removal of the medullary carcinoma can be monitored with serum calcitonin levels. Hyperparathyroidism, while unlikely in this patient, is probably present in his brother. These multiple adenomata are not associated with increased secretions of trophic hormones from the pituitary gland.

246. The answer is E. *(Felig, ed 2. pp 1415–1416.)* The clinical presentation of a bilateral pulmonary infiltrate, together with nephrocalcinosis, hypercalcemia, hyperuricemia, and normal phosphate levels, is typical of sarcoidosis. The absence of any bone lesion, together with a normal phosphate level, makes primary hyperparathyroidism unlikely. Furthermore, in primary hyperparathyroidism the serum chloride is frequently elevated and pulmonary infiltration, together with reduced vital capacity and diffusion defect, is uncharacteristic. The other causes of hypercalcemia are not associated with this clinical and biochemical constellation. The mechanism of hypercalcemia in sarcoidosis is not fully understood. It is thought that the hypercalcemia results from increased absorption of calcium from the gut, secondary to exaggerated vitamin D sensitivity. The mechanism for the reduction in hypercalcemia that follows steroid administration is unknown, but it is possible that glucocorticoids may inhibit formation of active vitamin D. To induce a remission, sarcoidosis is treated with prednisone, approximately 1 mg/kg per day.

247. The answer is E. *(Braunwald, ed 11. pp 1775–1778. Felig, ed 2. pp 667–672.)* Patients who have pheochromocytoma frequently demonstrate reduced circulating plasma volume, probably as a consequence of chronic, excessive alpha-adrenergic stimulation. Reduced plasma volume is suggested clinically by orthostatic hypotension or by elevated hematocrit. If plasma volume is reduced preoperatively and not corrected by infusion of plasma or treatment with phenoxybenzamine, severe hypotension may occur during surgery immediately after removal of the tumor. Hypotension under such circumstances is best treated with volume expansion (e.g., blood replacement) rather than with a vasoconstrictive agent.

248. The answer is A. *(Wilson, ed 7. pp 871–875.)* Congenital adrenal hyperplasia is characterized by an inherited enzymatic defect of steroidogenesis that interferes with the normal feedback inhibition of ACTH secretion, thus resulting in adrenal hyperplasia; it is an autosomal recessive disorder. Of the various enzyme deficiencies, only two, 11 β-hydroxylase and 17 α-hydroxylase deficiencies, are associated with hypertension. In 11 β-hydroxylase deficiency, the block creates a deficiency of cortisol, corticosterone, and aldosterone. The resultant accumulation of deoxycorticosterone protects against adrenal insufficiency and leads to salt and water retention, and the consequent volume expansion causes a suppression of renin activity. While men are only affected by hypertension, women also experience some degree of virilization due to excess androgen production. Treatment is with small doses of dexamethasone.

249. The answer is A. *(Braunwald, ed 11. pp 1751–1752.)* Although well-differentiated thyroid carcinomas in women under age 40 behave almost like benign disease, these tumors are far more aggressive in the elderly, particularly in men. Cold nodules are far less common in men than in women, and the risk of carcinoma is higher. Thus, the physician should not attempt a trial of suppressive thyroid treatment for a 60-year-old man who has a cold nodule, but should refer him for surgery. In such a patient, a needle biopsy could cause the tumor to spread and so should be avoided.

250. The answer is D. *(Braunwald, ed 11. pp 1250–1252.)* The diagnosis of gastrinoma should be considered in all patients with either recurrent ulcers after surgical correction for peptic ulcer disease, ulcers in the distal duodenum or jejunum, ulcer disease associated with diarrhea, or evidence suggestive of the MEN type I syndrome in ulcer patients. Because basal serum gastrin and basal acid production may both be normal or only slightly elevated in patients with gastrinomas, provocative tests may need to be employed for diagnosis. Both the secretin and calcium infusion tests are used; a paradoxical increase in serum gastrin concentration is seen in response to both infusions in patients with gastrinomas. In contrast, other conditions associated with hypergastrinemia such as duodenal ulcers, retained antrum, gastric outlet obstruction, antral G-cell hyperplasia, and pernicious anemia will respond with either no change or a decrease in serum gastrin.

251. The answer is D. *(Braunwald, ed 11. pp 1747–1748.)* Toxic multinodular goiter occurs not infrequently in a patient with long-standing simple goiter. This is a disease of the fifth or sixth decade of life, and women are affected much more frequently than men. The clinical presentation differs from that of typical Graves' disease. Exophthalmos is rare, while thyrotoxic cardiac disease is extremely common. Resistance to the usual therapeutic dosages of digitalis is common. The treatment of choice is radioactive iodine, and large doses, usually in excess of 20 μCi/g of estimated thyroid mass, are required. In order to prevent an exacerbation of thyrotoxic symptoms caused by the destruction of the thyroid gland and the release of thyroxine as a result of a radiation-induced thyroiditis, it is prudent to initiate therapy with antithyroid agents and administer the radioactive iodine as a definitive treatment only when the affected patient has become euthyroid. Propranolol is not required in euthyroid patients.

252. The answer is D. *(Braunwald, ed 11. pp 1822–1824, 1827. Felig, ed 2. pp 977–980.)* The failure of the patient presented in the question to respond to medroxyprogesterone acetate (Provera) indicates estrogen deficiency, while her ability to respond to estrogens rules out endometrial failure (e.g., Asherman's syndrome) as a basis for her disorder. Since patients who have psychiatric disorders and polycystic ovary syndromes continue to produce estrogens, they would be expected to exhibit both withdrawal bleeding after Provera and relatively normal production of gonadotropins. In the patient under discussion, a diagnosis of ovarian failure or premature menopause is indicated by the marked increase in gonadotropins. In contrast, patients suffering from pituitary tumors have reduced gonadotropins.

253. The answer is C. *(Braunwald, ed 11. pp 1574–1577. Felig, ed 2. pp 964–966.)* The symptoms of masculinization (e.g., alopecia, deepening of voice, clitoral hypertrophy) in the patient presented in the question are characteristic of active androgen-producing tumors. Such extreme virilization is very rarely observed in polycystic ovary syndrome or in Cushing's syndrome; moreover, the presence of normal urinary steroid and markedly elevated plasma testosterone levels indicates an ovarian rather than adrenal cause of her findings. Although hilar cell tumors are capable of producing the picture seen in this patient, they are very rare and usually arise in postmenopausal women. Arrhenoblastomas are the most common androgen-producing ovarian tumor. Their incidence is highest during the reproductive years. Composed of varying proportions of Leydig's and Sertoli's cells, they are generally benign. In contrast to arrhenoblastomas, granulosa-theca cell tumors produce feminization, not virilization.

254. The answer is D. *(Braunwald, ed 11. pp 1724–1729. Felig, ed 2. pp 357–368.)* Metastatic tumors rarely cause diabetes insipidus; of the tumors that may cause it, carcinoma of the breast is by far the most common. In the patient discussed in the question, the diagnosis of diabetes insipidus is suggested by hypernatremia and a low urine osmolality. Psychogenic polydipsia is an unlikely diagnosis since serum sodium is usually mildly reduced in this condition. Renal glycosuria would be expected to induce a higher urine osmolality than this patient has because of the osmotic effect of glucose. While nephrocalcinosis secondary to hypercalcemia may produce polyuria, hypercalciuria does not. Finally, the findings of inappropriate antidiuretic hormone syndrome are the opposite of those observed in diabetes insipidus and thus incompatible with the clinical picture in this patient.

255. The answer is C. *(Braunwald, ed 11. p 1741. Felig, ed 2. pp 76–77, 417.)* The patient presented in the question has a classic case of iodine-induced hypothyroidism (Wolff-Chaikoff effect). Normally, patients rapidly escape the suppressive effects of iodine on thyroid hormone production so that circulating thyroid hormone levels are unaffected. However, patients who are exposed to neck radiation (external or radioactive iodine) or who have glandular damage (thyroiditis or Graves' disease) are at risk of hypothyroidism. The source of iodine in this patient is the lymphangiogram, a procedure that would be expected to increase the patient's iodine pool for several years.

256. The answer is A (1, 2, 3). *(Wilson, ed 7. p 605.)* Hypersecretion of growth hormone is usually secondary to a somatotropic pituitary cell adenoma. Prior to epiphyseal closure, an increase in growth rate with minimal bony deformity is the common presentation; in adults, coarsening of facial features, soft tissue swelling of hands and feet, and bony proliferation are typical manifestations. Diagnosis rests on characteristics of growth hormone secretion that are unique to acromegalics. Random serum determinations range from normal to grossly elevated and in the vast majority of cases the sleep-related peak of growth hormone secretion is not found. While growth hormone levels are normally suppressed in response to a glucose load, levels may decrease, remain unchanged, or increase in 70 to 80 percent of patients; moreover, if suppressed, normal levels are never attained. An equally reliable finding is the increase in growth hormone seen after administration of TRH, a response not seen in normals. Because dopamine exerts an inhibitory effect on the adenoma, L-dopa, dopamine infusion, and morphine all suppress growth hormone levels in most acromegalics. While less useful as diagnostic aids, a paradoxical response to insulin-induced hypoglycemia and arginine infusion may be seen.

257. The answer is A (1, 2, 3). *(Braunwald, ed 11. pp 1843–1844.)* A number of defects may affect one of the X chromosomes of the female. The result is not only a failure to develop normal gonads but also the development of multiple congenital anomalies. Skeletal abnormalities may make diagnosis at birth possible, but more usually a failure to develop secondary sexual characteristics at puberty will draw attention to the problem. Although the genitalia are female, they remain immature and no breast development occurs. The inactivation of one of the X chromosomes produces the Barr body (sex chromatin) that can be used to screen for abnormalities of the X chromosome. Fifty percent of patients with Turner's syndrome (those who are 45,X) are chromatin-negative. In the remaining cases, karyotypic analysis is necessary not only to establish the diagnosis but to identify that subgroup of patients who have Y chromosomal elements present. Such patients have such a high incidence of malignancy developing in their primitive gonads that surgical removal is necessary. The management of this disease is based on supplying estrogen at the time of puberty to allow secondary sexual characteristics to develop and to help growth and bone maturation. Rarely do patients approach their predicted height. Unfortunately, the administration of growth hormone has not been able to influence the height achieved by these patients. Coarctation of the aorta is one of the anomalies seen in such patients; short fourth metacarpals are found in 50 percent of cases and the characteristic webbing of the neck is a prominent feature.

258. The answer is B (1, 3). *(Braunwald, ed 11. p 1748. Felig, ed 2. p 418.)* The clinical and laboratory findings in the patient presented in the question are most consistent with "T_3 toxicosis." This hyperthyroid state is a result of overproduction of triiodothyronine in the presence of normal or slightly elevated thyroxine. Radioactive iodine uptake may be normal or increased. "T_3 toxicosis" is observed most commonly in patients who have autonomous nodules or who have been treated for Graves' disease. The diagnosis is established either by the presence of elevated serum triiodothyronine (radioimmunoassay) or by an abnormal T_3 suppression test. In the patient presented, long-acting thyroid stimulator (LATS) would not be present; LATS is observed in Graves' disease but not in the presence of an autonomous nodule. While thyroid-stimulating hormone levels would be suppressed in this patient, currently the assay is not sensitive enough to distinguish between low normal values of this hormone and hyperthyroidism.

259. The answer is A (1, 2, 3). *(Wilson, ed 7. p 775.)* Thyroid storm is an acute exacerbation of partially treated or untreated thyrotoxicosis evoked by a precipitating factor such as infection, trauma, surgery, diabetic ketoacidosis, or pregnancy. The patient usually presents with fever, restlessness, nausea and vomiting, abdominal pain, tachycardia, diaphoresis, and, rarely, delirium. Treatment involves antagonizing all facets of thyroid hormone synthesis. Propylthiouracil, because it inhibits the iodination of tyrosine and monoiodotyrosine and prevents the coupling of iodotyrosines to form T_3 and T_4, is a first-line agent in the treatment of storm. As it also prevents the conversion of T_4 to T_3, it is preferred over methimazole, which does not affect this final step. Once iodination is inhibited, large doses of iodine are then administered in order to prevent the release of thyroid hormones. Dexamethasone, in addition to assuring adequate glucocorticoid stores, supports the actions of both propylthiouracil and iodine by inhibiting glandular release of hormone and preventing the conversion of T_4 to T_3. Propranolol is also given in order to reduce the effects of the increased sympathetic state.

260. The answer is D (4). *(Braunwald, ed 11. pp 1760–1764.)* While an abnormal diurnal steroid rhythm is a hallmark of Cushing's syndrome, it is a nonspecific finding and also may be observed in stress, obesity, or depression. Similarly, the overnight dexamethasone suppression test, virtually always abnormal in Cushing's syndrome, also may be abnormal in obesity, depression, severe illness, or in association with phenytoin (Dilantin) administration. Victims of Cushing's syndrome, in contrast to normal subjects, characteristically do not show an increase in blood cortisol after insulin-induced hypoglycemia. Finally, the presence of normal urinary 17-hydroxycorticosteroid excretion does not rule out the diagnosis of Cushing's syndrome; up to 15 percent of affected patients have values within normal limits.

261.   The answer is A (1, 2, 3). *(Braunwald, ed 11. pp 1724–1729. Felig, ed 2. pp 357–368.)* The ability of the patient presented in the question to concentrate urine clearly is impaired. His response to vasopressin (Pitressin) establishes the diagnosis of partial diabetes insipidus, thus ruling out psychogenic or nephrogenic causes for his urinary findings. Patients who have some antidiuretic hormone (ADH) secretion generally respond to oral chlorpropamide, thiazide diuretics, or lysine-vasopressin nasal spray. The negative salt balance induced by the diuretic leads to a reduction in glomerular filtration rate and to enhanced proximal tubular water reabsorption. This results in the delivery of less water to water-impermeable distal segments and so to reduced water excretion. While both chlorpropamide and tolbutamide have antidiuretic effects when given intravenously, only chlorpropamide is effective orally. The efficacy of sulfonylureas in this patient probably derives from their ability to enhance the action of ADH at the renal level.

262.   The answer is B (1, 3). *(Braunwald, ed 11. pp 1807–1811.)* Testicular function consists of two interrelated systems: one designed to produce sperm in spermatogenic tubules and the other to produce androgenic steroids, the most important of which is testosterone. These hormones are made in Leydig cells that are dispersed among the tubules. The major hormone regulating testosterone production is luteinizing hormone; follicle-stimulating hormone plays a less important role in the production of testosterone, but it is the major hormone regulating spermatogenesis. Male infertility can be associated with defects in both systems. Two syndromes have been identified that affect the cilia of the sperm, thus reducing their mobility and causing infertility. In Kartagener's syndrome the infertility is associated with situs inversus and the development of severe bronchiectasis. There is a defect in the protein dynein that is essential for the movement of both respiratory cilia and the sperm tail. In a second syndrome, this protein is normal but the radial spokes in the cilia are abnormal. Leydig cell function is assessed by obtaining plasma testosterone levels and, if they are low, exploring a pituitary cause for this defect by the simultaneous assay of plasma luteinizing hormone levels. Gonadotropin stimulation tests may be helpful. The measurement of urinary 17-ketosteroids is not helpful, as these androgens are mainly metabolites of hormones from the adrenal gland and testosterone is responsible for less than 40 percent of the daily production of 17-ketosteroids. The plasma levels of follicle-stimulating hormone can now be measured by a specific radioimmunoassay, and usually there is an inverse correlation between the levels and spermatogenesis. If the hypothalamic pituitary axis is normal, this hormone will be secreted in larger amounts after damage to the germinal epithelium of the Leydig cells.

263. The answer is C (2, 4). *(Braunwald, ed 11. pp 1707–1708. Felig, ed 2. p 619.)* Approximately 15 percent of patients who undergo bilateral adrenalectomy for Cushing's syndrome develop pituitary tumors that were not apparent prior to surgery (Nelson's syndrome); whether these tumors were actually present prior to surgery remains a point of speculation. Nelson's syndrome must be differentiated from inadequate adrenal replacement therapy, which will also produce hyperpigmentation. In either situation, circulating adrenocorticotropic hormone levels are increased.

264. The answer is C (2, 4). *(Braunwald, ed 11. pp 1871–1872. Felig, ed 2. pp 1379–1381.)* Hyperparathyroidism is frequently associated with personality changes, ranging from lethargy and mild affective disorders to mental obtundation and psychosis. The intensity of the symptoms is related to the magnitude of the hypercalcemia. Pruritus, which may be intense in hyperparathyroidism, disappears following parathyroidectomy. Electrocardiographic changes generally are limited to a shortening of the Q-T interval. Moniliasis is associated with hypoparathyroidism, not hyperparathyroidism.

265. The answer is E (all). *(Braunwald, ed 11. pp 1838–1840. Felig, ed 2. pp 886–889.)* Cirrhosis and uremia are among the most common causes of gynecomastia. Estrogen- and gonadotropin-secreting tumors and hypogonadism must also be considered as causes. In addition, exogenous estrogens, spironolactone, and digitalis may produce this abnormality. Gynecomastia occurs commonly during puberty, occasionally in association with hyperthyroidism, and after recovery from severe malnutrition.

266. The answer is C (2, 4). *(Braunwald, ed 11. pp 217–219. Spark, JAMA 243:750, 1980.)* Although psychological causes of impotence are responsible for the majority of cases, there are many drugs that have impotence as a side effect. Diuretics, methyldopa, and reserpine can produce complete or incomplete impotence. Recently it has been discovered that the widely used drugs cimetidine and spironolactone act as antiandrogens; in antagonizing the effects of androgen on the target tissue, they can affect the hormonal control of erection. While it is important to stress that the majority of patients taking these drugs do not suffer from impotence, physicians need to be aware of this possibility as these drugs have not been traditionally thought of in this context. Although clinical skills remain the best tools for sorting out the different causes of impotence, there are disturbances in endocrine function that may be responsible. Usually the measurement of plasma testosterone and prolactin in patients who have been consistently impotent for a period of more than 3 months will allow physicians to decide which patients have abnormalities of the endocrine system that require a more detailed evaluation. In one recent study of 105 patients presenting with impotence, 37 were found to have organic hypogonadism. Twenty of these patients had a hypothalamic pituitary deficiency. The incidence of impotence associated with antihypertensive treatment is as high as 17 percent.

267. The answer is B (1, 3). *(Braunwald, ed 11. p 1749.)* Thyrotoxicosis associated with decreased radioactive iodine (RAI) uptake has been observed in (1) patients who are surreptitiously taking exogenous thyroid; (2) Graves' disease with iodine loading; (3) iodine-induced thyrotoxicosis (jodbasedow phenomenon); (4) struma ovarii; and (5) metastatic follicular carcinoma. While a few rare cases of thyroid-stimulating hormone-producing pituitary adenomas have been reported, in this condition RAI uptake would be increased. Oat-cell carcinoma is associated with several ectopic hormone syndromes but not with thyroid overproduction.

268. The answer is E (all). *(Braunwald, ed 11. pp 1708–1717.)* Enlargement of the sella turcica is characteristic, but not diagnostic, of pituitary tumors. Suprasellar lesions like craniopharyngiomas and aneurysms may extend into the sella, producing enlargement of the sella and erosion of its walls. In addition, cerebrospinal fluid pressure can force the subarachnoid space into the sella, resulting in enlargement of the sella and compression of the normal pituitary (empty-sella syndrome).

269. The answer is A (1, 2, 3). *(Braunwald, ed 11. pp 1788–1790.)* Acetoacetate levels—in contrast to glucose, β-hydroxybutyrate, and free fatty acid levels—may actually rise during the first few hours of insulin treatment for diabetic ketoacidosis. Since Acetest tablets and Ketostix measure acetoacetate rather than β-hydroxybutyrate (the major blood ketone), such serial measurements of serum ketones do not reflect the blood ketone response to treatment. For example, total blood ketones, as measured by quantitative enzymatic techniques, may decline by 50 percent during the first few hours of treatment without a demonstrable change in serum ketones, as measured by Acetest tablets and Ketostix.

270. The answer is B (1, 3). *(Braunwald, ed 11. pp 1760–1764. Felig, ed 2. p 608.)* Regardless of pathogenesis, Cushing's syndrome is characterized by excess production of cortisol. Most cases are due to bilateral adrenal hyperplasia secondary to overproduction of ACTH by the pituitary. Harvey Cushing originally suggested (1932) that the excess ACTH was produced by pituitary basophil adenomas, a condition that was designated Cushing's disease before it was recognized that pituitary basophilism was only one of the causes of the syndrome that would bear his name. Because tumors may be very small and elude detection, or not be present at all, the frequency of pituitary adenomas as the cause of Cushing's syndrome is uncertain. The 48-hour dexamethasone suppression test is still an important screening test, since the failure of suppression of urinary 17-hydroxysteroid levels to less than

3 mg/24 hours, or of plasma cortisol levels to less than 5 μg/100 ml, by this test is virtually diagnostic of the syndrome. The most common nonendocrine tumor that secretes ACTH is a small-cell (oat-cell) carcinoma of the lung. In this situation, or in patients with adrenal neoplasms, no suppression occurs after dexamethasone administration, since pituitary ACTH secretion is already suppressed by the elevated cortisol levels. While routine laboratory examinations are rarely of major diagnostic utility in the diagnosis of Cushing's syndrome, certain abnormalities are suggestive: high normal values of hemoglobin, hematocrit, and red-cell count; a total lymphocyte count below normal in 35 percent of patients, and an eosinophil count usually below 100/mm^3; and fasting hyperglycemia in 10 to 15 percent of patients.

271. The answer is B (1, 3). *(Braunwald, ed 11. pp 1791–1792.)* The earliest sign of retinal change in diabetes is increased permeability followed by occlusion of retinal capillaries with sacular and fusiform aneurysms. Two types of exudates occur: (1) cotton wool exudates, or microinfarcts, and (2) hard exudates. A sudden increase in the number of cotton wool exudates suggests rapidly advancing retinopathy. Hard exudates are much more common than cotton wool exudates. These lesions are probably indicative of leakage of lipids, serum, and protein through damaged endothelium.

272. The answer is B (1, 3). *(Braunwald, ed 11. pp 1027, 1764, 1766. Felig, ed 2. pp 751–764.)* Diuretic therapy and malignant hypertension often induce excessive secretion of renin leading to secondary hyperaldosteronism, a condition that may be distinguished from primary hyperaldosteronism by elevated levels of renin. Renin is characteristically suppressed in primary hyperaldosteronism. Aldosterone levels are normal or low in Cushing's syndrome; hypokalemia in this disorder results from excessive cortisol and deoxycorticosterone production. Excessive licorice ingestion may produce hypokalemia and hypertension because of glycyrrhizic acid in the licorice. This mineralocorticoid-like substance expands plasma volume and reduces aldosterone secretion.

273. The answer is A (1, 2, 3). *(Braunwald, ed 11. p 1877. Felig, ed 2. pp 1415–1416.)* The association of hypercalcemia with sarcoidosis is often most striking in summer and, in fact, may disappear in winter. This fluctuation probably is mediated by the effects of sunlight on vitamin D synthesis. Characteristically, patients who have sarcoidosis, vitamin D intoxication, or malignancy demonstrate a fall in serum calcium after cortisone treatment (100 to 200 mg/day). Parathormone levels in hypercalcemic disorders not associated with hyperparathyroidism characteristically are low. Brown tumors are associated with hyperparathyroidism and represent areas of uncalcified bone; they are not observed in sarcoidosis.

274. The answer is B (1, 3). *(Braunwald, ed 11. pp 1871–1872. Felig, ed 2. pp 1384–1388.)* Although symptomatic bone disease is uncommon in hyperparathyroidism, affected patients with asymptomatic bone involvement may exhibit early x-ray changes, among the earliest of which are subperiosteal resorption of the phalanges and resorption of the phalangeal tufts. X-ray evidence of hyperparathyroidism elsewhere in the skeleton without abnormal hand x-rays is unusual. Osteosclerosis is observed in hypoparathyroidism, and pseudofractures appear in osteomalacia.

275. The answer is D (4). *(Braunwald, ed 11. pp 1747–1748. Felig, ed 2. pp 422–423.)* Onycholysis, or distal separation of the nail bed, is observed in over 10 percent of patients who have hyperthyroidism resulting from either Graves' disease or toxic nodular goiter; it usually begins in the nail of the fourth finger. In contrast, pretibial myxedema and exophthalmos are virtually pathognomonic of Graves' disease and are not observed in patients who have toxic nodular goiter. Thyroid acropathy, almost always associated with a history of exophthalmos and Graves' disease, is characterized by clubbing of the fingers and toes, swelling of the subcutaneous tissues of the extremities, and subperiosteal bone changes without new bone formation.

276. The answer is E (all). *(Braunwald, ed 11. pp 1837–1838.)* Numerous endocrine interactions are required for the letdown phenomenon that establishes milk flow. Clearly, prolactin is a major hormone involved in this process. However, in women who have not been pregnant or in men, the presence of high levels of prolactin in the serum is not sufficient to cause a secretion of milk. A number of cases of galactorrhea appear to be mild and idiopathic, but it is important to remember that pituitary tumors have been found in patients many months after an initial work-up for a pituitary lesion was negative. The higher the prolactin values and the more troublesome the galactorrhea, the more likely it is that a pituitary tumor will eventually be found. Interruption of the pituitary stalk produces a striking increase in prolactin secretion because of the unavailability to the pituitary gland of prolactin inhibitory factor. A number of drugs seem to have the same effect. Examples are alpha methyldopa, reserpine, antiemetics, and most psychotropic agents. The central role of prolactin in the production of galactorrhea is probably best demonstrated by the therapeutic efficacy of bromocriptine mesylate. This agent is very successful in blocking the secretion of milk, which it does by suppressing plasma prolactin levels. In those women whose galactorrhea is complicated by amenorrhea, this drug may serve a dual purpose: blocking milk production and stimulating the resumption of normal menstrual cycles.

277. The answer is A (1, 2, 3). *(Braunwald, ed 11. pp 1795–1796. Felig, ed 2. pp 1416–1417.)* Patients who are restricted to total bedrest or subject to stress will demonstrate glucose intolerance that is a consequence of insulin resistance. Furthermore, immobilization of young patients undergoing rapid bone growth can result in hypercalcemia and hypercalciuria. The hypercalcemia, in turn, will suppress parathyroid secretion. The severe pain and stress of a fracture, such as in the boy presented in the question, could lead to the loss of normal diurnal rhythm for cortisol secretion.

278. The answer is C (2, 4). *(Braunwald, ed 11. pp 1724–1729.)* The response to dehydration provides the most simple and reliable way for establishing the diagnosis of diabetes insipidus. Fluid is usually withheld from 6 A.M. to allow the patient to be carefully monitored over a sufficiently long period of time. It is necessary to withhold fluids until stable hourly urinary osmolalities have been established. A loss of body weight of approximately 1 kg will usually accompany this degree of fluid deprivation. A loss of greater than 2 kg of body weight would be hazardous to the patient and fluid deprivation must be discontinued at this point. Generally, 5 units of vasopressin tannate in oil is given subcutaneously a few hours after dehydration is started, with serum osmolality being determined immediately before the injection of vasopressin and urinary osmolality being carefully monitored during the hour that follows the injection. Until recently, the most effective treatment of diabetes insipidus had been to supply arginine vasopressin, which has a duration of action from 4 to 6 hours and could be administered as an intranasal snuff. However, a new synthetic vasopressin, desmopressin acetate (DDAVP), is the preferred drug for the management of diabetes insipidus because a single dose has a duration of action from 12 to 24 hours. A number of diuretics have been paradoxically successful in preventing the loss of fluids in diabetes insipidus, of which hydrochlorothiazide and chlorthalidone are the most successful. Ethacrynic acid, however, is not effective. The tranquilizer thioridazine (Mellaril) can produce a syndrome of water intoxication with normal diluting capacity in patients with diabetes insipidus. Similar toxicity has been noted in patients who have required large enemas or who have drunk large volumes of beer. Other drugs that have been useful in the management of diabetes insipidus include the sulfonylurea chlorpropamide, which has been shown to stimulate ADH release from the neurohypophysis, and the anticholesterol drug clofibrate.

279. The answer is A (1, 2, 3). *(Braunwald, ed 11. pp 1738, 1741.)* More than 95 percent of patients who have Hashimoto's thyroiditis demonstrate high titers of thyroglobulin antibodies, thyroid microsomal antibodies, or both. Extremely high titers are virtually diagnostic of the disease. Lower titers of thyroid antibodies may be observed in 50 percent of patients afflicted with pernicious anemia and in 20 percent of elderly women. Relatives of patients suffering from Hashimoto's or Graves' disease, as well as patients who have other autoimmune diseases, also exhibit low titers of thyroid antibody.

280. The answer is E (all). *(Braunwald, ed 11. pp 1749–1750.)* Subacute thyroiditis is characterized by acute or subacute onset of asthenia, malaise, and pain over the thyroid that often is referred to the ear, lower jaw, or occiput. The disease is probably viral in origin; it frequently follows an upper respiratory infection. Subacute thyroiditis is diagnosed on the basis of an elevated erythrocyte sedimentation rate and a markedly depressed radioactive iodine uptake. Frequently, a high serum T_4 level is observed, which, together with "leakage" of iodine from the gland, produces an elevated protein-bound iodine level.

281. The answer is B (1, 3). *(Braunwald, ed 11. pp 1900–1902. Felig, ed 2. pp 1483–1491.)* Paget's disease is characterized by excessive and abnormal remodeling of bone. The markedly increased bone turnover leads to elevations in serum alkaline phosphatase level and in urine hydroxyproline excretion. Serum and urinary calcium levels are normal; however, during periods of immobilization, patients afflicted with Paget's disease can develop severe hypercalcemia and hypercalciuria.

282–285. The answers are: 282-D, 283-C, 284-A, 285-B. *(Braunwald, ed 11. pp 1703, 1729–1731, 1761, 1767–1769. Felig, ed 2. pp 599–620, 1692–1698.)* Ectopic adrenocorticotropic hormone (ACTH) syndrome, as may be caused by oat-cell carcinoma, is characterized by hypokalemic alkalosis, hyperpigmentation associated with elevated levels of ACTH, and myopathy. The characteristic clinical features of Cushing's syndrome are generally absent, probably because of the rapid development of the disorder. Urinary 17-hydroxycorticosteroids (OHCS) and 17-ketosteroids (KS), as well as plasma cortisol, are markedly elevated; dexamethasone fails to suppress 17-OHCS even when high doses are given.

Cushing's syndrome (bilateral adrenal hyperplasia) is characterized by the loss of diurnal variation in plasma cortisol, elevated urinary 17-OHCS, the failure of urinary 17-OHCS suppression with the low-dose dexamethasone test, and greater than 50 percent suppression with the high-dose dexamethasone test. Plasma ACTH concentration is normal or mildly elevated and hypokalemic alkalosis is rarely present. Urinary 17-KS levels may be normal or increased inasmuch as they do not reflect the rate of cortisol production.

Patients who have adrenal carcinoma often display signs of excess adrenal androgen production that sometimes overshadow the signs of Cushing's syndrome. Plasma cortisol and urinary 17-KS may be dramatically increased; there is no 17-OHCS or 17-KS suppression even with the high-dose dexamethasone test. Characteristically, in adrenal carcinoma plasma ACTH is very low; in contrast, in Cushing's syndrome and ectopic ACTH syndrome, the ACTH levels are normal or increased.

Congenital adrenal hyperplasia results from a deficiency of one of several possible cortisol synthetic enzymes, the most common being 21-hydroxylase. Adrenal androgen production often is dramatically increased, while adrenal cortisol production may be normal or decreased. As a consequence of the excess androgen production, virilism occurs in the female and short stature is frequent in the male because of early closure of bony epiphyses. Urinary 17-KS levels are increased in congenital adrenal hyperplasia but are suppressed by dexamethasone. This feature distinguishes the disorder from adrenal tumors. Hyperpigmentation results from the compensatory increase in ACTH secretion.

286–289. The answers are: 286-C, 287-A, 288-B, 289-D. *(Braunwald, ed 11. pp 1650–1661. Felig, ed 2. pp 1245–1280.)* "Broad-beta" disease is characterized by the accumulation of remnants of abnormal, very-low-density lipoproteins (VLDL). These remnants, displaying a mobility on lipoprotein electrophoresis between prebeta- and betalipoproteins, present as a broad smear (''broad-beta band'') between those two lipoprotein zones. On ultracentrifugation, however, the remnants sediment with VLDL. Plasma triglycerides and cholesterol are present in an approximate 1:1 ratio. The disorder is familial and associated with premature vascular disease. Planar xanthomas and tuberoeruptive xanthomas (confluent, eruptive lesions) of the elbows are virtually pathognomonic of ''broad-beta'' disease.

Hyperchylomicronemia results from lipoprotein lipase deficiency. This is a familial disorder that usually appears in childhood, producing recurrent abdominal pain, pancreatitis, and signs of extreme elevations of triglycerides. The chylomicron test will show a thick creamy layer on top and clear plasma below.

Hyperbetalipoproteinemia is inherited as a dominant trait. Afflicted heterozygous individuals generally develop ischemic heart disease before the fifth decade of life. Clinical features include tendinous and tuberous xanthomas, arcus corneae, and, occasionally, xanthelasma. The presumptive metabolic defect in this disorder is a defect in betalipoprotein removal.

Hyperprebetalipoproteinemia may be familial but is more commonly secondary to another cause (e.g., alcohol, stress, diabetes mellitus, uremia, obesity, glucocorticoids, or estrogens). In the case of estrogens, increases in triglycerides are secondary to increased VLDL production.

290–294. The answers are: 290-B, 291-C, 292-B, 293-A, 294-A. *(Wilson, ed 7. pp 1274–1283.)* The components of MEN I are hyperparathyroidism, pancreatic islet cell tumors, and anterior pituitary tumors; tumors of the adrenal cortex and thyroid are less frequent features. The syndrome is inherited in an autosomal dominant fashion and presentations occur at any age. While asymptomatic hypercalcemia is common, 50 percent of patients have renal stones and 25 percent have osteitis fibrosa as manifestations of hyperparathyroidism. Most pancreatic islet cell tumors secrete gastrin or insulin and 10 percent of patients have complications of both. The diagnosis of gastrinomas rests on the demonstration of increased gastrin levels after secretin infusion, while insulinomas are characterized by fasting hypoglycemia coexistent with an elevated plasma insulin level. Pituitary tumors present either because of their size or because of their secretory capabilities; prolactinomas are the most common tumor type.

MEN II, in contrast, is characterized by medullary thyroid carcinoma, pheochromocytoma, and hyperparathyroidism; it is also transmitted in autosomal dominant fashion. Glandular involvement is typically multicentric as it is in MEN I. Metastatic thyroid carcinoma is associated with early metastatic disease and multiple secretory products, the most common of which is calcitonin. Pheochromocytoma, the major cause of morbidity and mortality in patients with MEN II, typically develops at an older age and occurs as bilateral adrenal tumors in 60 to 70 percent of cases. These tumors manifest as hypertension and paroxysms of flushing, sweating, and headaches, or they may be asymptomatic. They are diagnosed by finding increased levels of catecholamines or catecholamine metabolites in a 24-hour urine collection. Unlike patients with MEN I, most patients with MEN II and parathyroid hyperplasia are normocalcemic.

295–299. The answers are: 295-A, 296-C, 297-C, 298-D, 299-D. *(Felig, ed 2. pp 432–435.)* Hyperthyroidism results from the excessive secretion of thyroid hormones and is most commonly due to Graves' disease, thyroiditis, multinodular goiter, or thyroid adenoma. The choice of therapy, whether with antithyroid drugs, radiation, or surgery, is influenced by the patient's age and sex, status of the hyperthyroidism and cardiovascular system, and history of previous management of the disease.

The thionamide drugs used in the United States are propylthiouracil (PTU) and methimazole. Both drugs inhibit the incorporation of iodide into thyroglobulin by blocking iodine oxidation and organification and iodotyrosine coupling. They do not, however, block the release of previously formed and stored thyroid hormone. PTU has the advantage of inhibiting the extrathyroidal conversion of T_4 to T_3. Both drugs also have immunosuppressive activity: thyroid antibody production is inhibited, as are lymphocyte function and viability.

While the plasma half-life of PTU is 1 to 2 hours and that of methimazole is 4 to 6 hours, because the drugs are concentrated in the thyroid gland, serum levels do not reflect intrathyroidal concentrations.

Toxic reactions to these drugs occur in 5 to 10 percent of patients and most commonly consist of pruritus, urticaria, and other rashes; more serious side effects include fever, arthritis, vasculitis, hepatitis, anemia, and thrombocytopenia. In 0.5 percent of patients, a rapidly developing agranulocytosis occurs.

Gastroenterology

DIRECTIONS: Each question below contains five suggested responses. Select the **one best** response to each question.

300. A physician is investigating a patient with a clinical condition compatible with malabsorption. In his attempts to differentiate between a primary malabsorptive defect and impaired digestion (e.g., pancreatic insufficiency), he orders a number of tests. All the following information about such tests is accurate EXCEPT that

(A) quantitation of stool fat will not help distinguish pancreatic insufficiency from nontropical sprue
(B) lactase deficiency can be diagnosed accurately by measuring hydrogen excreted in the breath after a loading dose of lactose
(C) the triolein absorption test is normal in malabsorption syndromes, except those involving pancreatic insufficiency
(D) measurement of serum carotenes provides a satisfactory but nondiscriminate screening test for malabsorption
(E) unless there is bacterial overgrowth, analysis of duodenal fluid for conjugated bile salts will not reveal an abnormality in either nontropical sprue or pancreatic insufficiency

301. A 55-year-old man with a several-year history of reflux esophagitis is found on esophagoscopy and biopsy to have the distal esophagus lined by columnar epithelium. True statements regarding this patient's condition include all the following EXCEPT

(A) scintigraphic scanning with ^{99m}Tc pertechnetate is a reliable diagnostic test for this condition
(B) the use of antacids results in symptomatic improvement
(C) frequent endoscopies with multiple biopsies and cytologic examinations should be recommended
(D) strictures are typically found in mid-esophagus
(E) no regression of the histologic abnormality occurs with either antacid or cimetidine therapy

302. Acute pancreatitis is best characterized by which of the following statements?

(A) The amylase/creatinine clearance ratio is usually less than 1
(B) The degree of elevation in serum amylase is a relatively accurate index of the clinical severity of the lesion
(C) It is generally accepted that the development of a pancreatic pseudocyst is an indication for immediate surgical intervention with internal drainage
(D) Types I and V hyperlipidemias are predisposing factors
(E) Hypoglycemia, as a result of deficient glucagon levels, is a relatively common manifestation

303. A 45-year-old woman with a long history of heavy drinking is admitted to the hospital because of weakness, anorexia, abdominal pain, and fatigue. On examination, she is found to have significant hepatomegaly, jaundice, ascites, and splenomegaly. Which of the following laboratory findings is LEAST likely in this patient?

(A) Greatly elevated serum γ-glutamyl transpeptidase
(B) Greatly elevated serum IgA
(C) Absent prebetalipoprotein band with all lipoproteins migrating as a single wide band
(D) Smooth muscle antibody present in a titer of 1:100
(E) Hyperuricemia

304. All the following are possible complications of jejunoileal bypass surgery EXCEPT

(A) polyarthritis
(B) diarrhea
(C) nephrolithiasis
(D) electrolyte imbalance
(E) chronic active hepatitis

305. All the following statements about idiopathic hemochromatosis are true EXCEPT that

(A) the disorder is inherited as an autosomal recessive trait
(B) the disorder has an association with HLA-A3
(C) in untreated patients with clinically manifest hemochromatosis, serum ferritin level correlates with the magnitude of body iron stores
(D) in established cases, weekly phlebotomy reduces iron stores to normal within 6 months
(E) following reduction of iron stores to normal, phlebotomy is required every 3 to 4 months to prevent reaccumulation of iron

306. A 25-year-old woman develops severe pruritus during the last trimester of her first pregnancy. She is mildly jaundiced. Within 2 weeks of delivery, both pruritus and jaundice disappear. All the following statements concerning this patient's symptoms are true EXCEPT that

(A) they will recur with subsequent pregnancies
(B) they usually occur throughout the course of a pregnancy
(C) they may be reproduced if the patient takes birth control pills
(D) they may have a genetic predisposition
(E) in the presence of symptoms, liver biopsy will show only mild cholestasis

307. A 40-year-old man has symptoms suggestive of a peptic ulcer. An upper GI series reveals a small, apparently uncomplicated duodenal ulcer. In addition, there is marked rugal hypertrophy in the stomach and swelling of the folds in the duodenum. The next step in the evaluation of this patient should be

(A) panendoscopy
(B) gastric analysis
(C) assay of serum gastrin
(D) pancreatic function tests
(E) barium enema

308. Ulcerative colitis is associated with all the following complications EXCEPT

(A) ankylosing spondylitis
(B) arthritis of the large joints
(C) clubbing of the fingers
(D) erythema multiforme
(E) hepatocellular carcinoma

309. A 34-year-old man presents with a 3-month history of hematochezia, tenesmus, and a vague abdominal discomfort. On sigmoidoscopy, a glistening, edematous, and hyperemic mucosa is seen, which bleeds easily after being touched, is limited to the distal 7 cm of rectum, and is sharply demarcated from the normal bowel above. The differential diagnosis includes all the following EXCEPT

(A) salmonellosis
(B) shigellosis
(C) giardiasis
(D) amebiasis
(E) gonorrhea

310. A 60-year-old man known to have colonic diverticulosis presents with rectal hemorrhage, requiring a transfusion of 2 units of blood. Which of the following statements is most likely to apply to this patient's situation?

(A) Hemorrhage as a result of diverticular disease almost always is associated with inflamed diverticula
(B) Bleeding from diverticula usually ceases spontaneously and conservative management generally suffices
(C) Bleeding is relatively uncommon because the diverticula usually form on the antimesenteric border, away from the blood vessels
(D) Colonoscopy frequently fails to reveal the bleeding diverticula
(E) The presence of diverticulosis increases the likelihood of colonic carcinoma

311. A 50-year-old alcoholic woman undergoes an upper gastrointestinal series to evaluate vague, dyspeptic symptoms, and a loss of weight. She is found to have a small ulcer on the greater curvature of the stomach. The ulcer is sharply punched out, exhibiting radiating folds and Hampton's line. All the following statements in reference to this patient are correct EXCEPT that

(A) gastroscopy and biopsy should be performed
(B) gastric acid studies are useful only if absolute achlorhydria is found
(C) if the ulcer is benign, there is a 50 percent chance that it will heal in 3 weeks and a 70 percent chance that it will heal in 6 weeks
(D) if the ulcer is benign, a repeat upper GI series should be done at 8 weeks with recommendation for surgery if the ulcer has not healed
(E) alcohol seems to play a role in the development of gastritis

312. A 45-year-old man develops dark urine, pale stools, nausea, anorexia, and upper right quadrant discomfort. On examination, his liver is found to be palpable two finger-breadths below the costal margin with a total span of 17 cm; the spleen is palpable below the costal margin and the abdomen exhibits shifting dullness. The patient indicates that he drinks 3 to 4 ounces or more of gin a day. In addition, he had eaten raw clams 3 weeks before the onset of his symptoms. For the past 3 years he has been taking alpha methyldopa (Aldomet) for hypertension. Serologic screening reveals the presence of hepatitis A antibody (IgG), anti-HBs (titer: 1:16 by RIA), and anti-HBc (titer: 1:8 by RIA). Other laboratory values are as follows:

Bilirubin, total, serum: 10.5 mg/100 ml
Bilirubin, direct, serum: 6.7 mg/100 ml
SGOT: 94 IU/L
SGPT: 42 IU/L
Alkaline phosphatase, serum: 200 U/L

The most likely diagnosis is

(A) acute hepatitis A
(B) acute hepatitis B
(C) non-A, non-B hepatitis
(D) alcoholic hepatitis
(E) drug-induced hepatitis related to alpha methyldopa

313. A healthy 22-year-old man is found to have a total serum bilirubin level of 2.5 mg/100 ml, with a direct fraction of 0.1 mg/100 ml. Other liver function tests are normal, and there is no evidence of hemolysis. The serum bilirubin level in this patient will undergo which of the following changes?

(A) Increase with phenobarbital therapy
(B) Gradually increase as he becomes older
(C) Increase during a 24-hour fast
(D) Diminish with high protein feeding
(E) Decrease after heavy exercise

314. A 76-year-old man complains to his physician that for 6 months he has developed regularly severe abdominal pain 1 to 2 hours after eating. So bad is the pain that he is losing weight because he is afraid to eat. There is no blood in his stool. The most likely diagnosis for his problem is

(A) diverticulosis
(B) regional enteritis
(C) irritable bowel syndrome
(D) mesenteric angina
(E) amyloidosis

315. In an alcoholic patient, the clinical or historical finding that has the best prognostic correlation with the development of cirrhosis is

(A) liver biopsy evidence of alcoholic hepatitis
(B) the degree of fatty infiltration on liver biopsy
(C) the level of serum glutamic oxaloacetic transaminase
(D) the nutritional status of the affected patient
(E) the type of liquor imbibed

316. A 44-year-old man complains of colicky abdominal pain, dark urine, and light stools of 1 week's duration. On examination, he is found to have moderate hepatomegaly, the hepatic edge being felt 4 cm below the costal margin. The gallbladder is not palpable, and there are no other abnormalities. Laboratory values are as follows:

Bilirubin, total, serum: 10.4 mg/100 ml
Bilirubin, direct, serum: 6.9 mg/100 ml
SGOT: 90 IU/L
Alkaline phosphatase, serum: 270 IU/L (normal: 21 to 91)

The results of a cholangiographic study appear in the x-ray below. The most likely diagnosis is

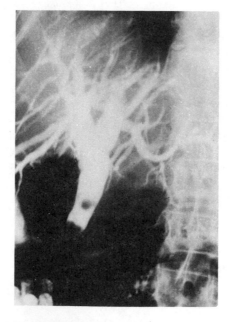

(A) carcinoma of the head of the pancreas
(B) carcinoma of the common bile duct
(C) carcinoma of the ampulla of Vater
(D) stone in the common duct
(E) stone in the cystic duct

317. All the following statements about parenteral feeding are true EXCEPT that

(A) patients receiving central vein feedings should have their urine and blood glucose monitored on a daily basis

(B) when the goal of central feeding is weight gain, the infusions should aim to provide 7000 kcal/week in excess of metabolic requirements

(C) hospitalized patients who have rapidly lost more than 10 percent of their body weight should be considered for parenteral feeding

(D) linoleic and linolenic acids are two polyunsaturated fatty acids that cannot be synthesized and must be supplied in a parenteral diet

(E) feeding via peripheral veins is limited, as the requirements for isotonicity make it impossible to deliver 2300 kcal in less than 3 L

318. A 35-year-old woman complains of weight loss and frequent, greasy, foul-smelling stools. She is observed to have thickened skin on her hands with ulcerations of the fingertips. Her gastrointestinal condition should be treated with

(A) surgery
(B) steroids
(C) azathioprine
(D) tetracycline
(E) gamma globulin injections

319. A 38-year-old woman was recovering from a viral flu-like illness with bed rest and aspirin for her symptoms. She was improving when quite suddenly she developed severe intractable vomiting. She rapidly became dehydrated and confused and lapsed into a coma. She was admitted to a hospital, where seizure activity required therapy. Apart from mild hepatomegaly, no other abnormalities were found on physical examination. Liver enzymes were increased in her serum, as was the concentration of ammonia. The most likely diagnosis in this condition is

(A) Reye's syndrome
(B) leptospirosis
(C) equine encephalitis
(D) disseminated cytomegalovirus infection
(E) poisoning by the wild mushroom *Amanita phalloides*

DIRECTIONS: Each question below contains four suggested responses of which **one or more** is correct. Select

A	if	**1, 2, and 3**	are correct
B	if	**1 and 3**	are correct
C	if	**2 and 4**	are correct
D	if	**4**	is correct
E	if	**1, 2, 3, and 4**	are correct

320. A 48-year-old woman complains of a 2-month history of intermittent right upper quadrant aching, jaundice, and pruritus. Subsequent cholangiography reveals thickened bile duct walls with narrow, beaded lumina. True statements concerning this condition include that

(1) it is attended by a mean survival of 4 to 10 years
(2) portal hypertension is a common complication
(3) a search for inflammatory bowel disease should be made
(4) corticosteroid therapy is efficacious

321. An elevated level of breath hydrogen after ingestion of 50 g of lactose is associated with which of the following conditions?

(1) Tropical sprue
(2) Ulcerative colitis
(3) Giardiasis
(4) Abetalipoproteinemia

322. True statements concerning granulomatous hepatitis include that

(1) sarcoidosis is the most common cause
(2) viral infections have been shown to cause hepatic granulomata
(3) histologic resolution follows successful therapy
(4) hyperbilirubinemia is a frequent finding

323. True statements concerning pancreatic abscesses complicating pancreatitis include

(1) they are often multiple
(2) they commonly occur within the first week after presentation
(3) they are usually polymicrobial
(4) antibiotic therapy is curative in the majority of patients

324. True statements concerning achalasia include which of the following?

(1) Patients frequently present with chest pain
(2) While lower esophageal pressure is increased, peristalsis remains normal
(3) Liquids typically do not cause dysphagia
(4) It is associated with an increased incidence of esophageal carcinoma

325. The Budd-Chiari syndrome, a condition involving hepatic venous outflow obstruction, is characterized by

(1) a lower-than-normal radioisotope uptake in the caudate lobe of the liver together with increased uptake in the right lobe
(2) a frequently successful response to a side-to-side portacaval shunt procedure
(3) a histologic appearance featuring peliosis hepatis in liver biopsy specimens
(4) severe ascites that is resistant to therapy

326. Correct statements about primary biliary cirrhosis, a chronic disease characterized by progressive ductular damage, include which of the following?

(1) Gallstones are more common in affected patients than in the general population
(2) Penicillamine effectively limits both the degree of ductular damage and the development of overt portal hypertension
(3) Pruritus almost always precedes jaundice
(4) The female:male ratio of occurrence is about 3:1

327. A 57-year-old man has clinical and histologic evidence of chronic active hepatitis. His serum is positive for HBsAg. Antigens and antibodies that are likely to be found by radioimmunoassay in the serum of this patient include

(1) HBeAg
(2) Anti-HBc
(3) Anti-HA (IgG)
(4) Anti-HBs

328. Non-A, non-B hepatitis is the most important form of posttransfusion hepatitis. Correct statements concerning non-A, non-B hepatitis include which of the following?

(1) Nonparenteral transmission occurs in a significant number of affected patients
(2) Anicteric hepatitis is as common as icteric hepatitis
(3) Gamma globulin given immediately after exposure has not been shown to reduce significantly the total incidence of hepatitis
(4) Chronic active hepatitis commonly follows this infection, has a more fulminant course than hepatitis B, and has a higher long-term mortality

SUMMARY OF DIRECTIONS

A	B	C	D	E
1,2,3 only	1,3 only	2,4 only	4 only	All are correct

329. Acute stress ulceration is a common complication in critically ill patients whose major illness relates to another organ system. True statements regarding stress erosions include

(1) the majority bleed
(2) an increase in overall mortality has been shown with even nonbleeding gastric mucosal injury
(3) they usually occur in the locations of typical peptic ulcers
(4) severe head injuries are a risk factor in their development

330. A middle-aged woman presents complaining of a 9-month history of diarrhea, weight loss, abdominal pain, and increased skin pigmentation. Biopsy of the small intestine reveals an overwhelming number of foamy, PAS-positive macrophages in the lamina propria. Correct statements about this patient's condition include which of the following?

(1) Steroids are contraindicated
(2) It is typically associated with a deforming polyarthritis
(3) A pigmented buccal mucosa is characteristic
(4) Focal cranial nerve signs may be present

331. Correct statements about Wilson's disease include which of the following?

(1) While patients with Wilson's disease may have normal levels of ceruloplasmin, low levels are diagnostic
(2) It may present as a Coombs-positive hemolytic anemia
(3) Duration of therapy with penicillamine averages 3 to 5 years
(4) Proper treatment prevents virtually all manifestations of the disease

332. Small bowel bacterial overgrowth may lead to which of the following complications?

(1) Vitamin B_{12} deficiency
(2) Steatorrhea
(3) Protein losing enteropathy
(4) Folate deficiency

DIRECTIONS: Each group of questions below consists of four lettered headings followed by a set of numbered items. For each numbered item select

A	if the item is associated with	(A) **only**
B	if the item is associated with	(B) **only**
C	if the item is associated with	**both** (A) and (B)
D	if the item is associated with	**neither** (A) nor (B)

Each lettered heading may be used **once, more than once, or not at all.**

Questions 333–337

(A) Chronic active hepatitis
(B) Chronic persistent hepatitis
(C) Both
(D) Neither

333. Relapses with discontinuation of corticosteroids

334. Acute onset typical

335. Ulcerative colitis

336. Piecemeal necrosis typical on liver biopsy

337. Methyldopa

Questions 338–342

(A) Familial polyposis coli (colonic polyposis)
(B) Gardner's syndrome
(C) Both
(D) Neither

338. Imperative screening of family members by sigmoidoscopy and barium enema

339. Congenital hypertrophy of retinal pigment epithelium

340. Osteomas of jaw and skull

341. Indication for prophylactic colectomy

342. Multiple hamartomatous polyps of the entire gastrointestinal tract

Questions 343–347

(A) Serum glutamic oxaloacetic transaminase (SGOT)
(B) Serum glutamic pyruvic transaminase (SGPT)
(C) Both
(D) Neither

343. Level of elevation correlates with extent of liver necrosis on biopsy

344. Elevations are typically less than 500 IU in alcoholic hepatitis

345. Levels are usually greater than 1000 IU in extrahepatic obstruction

346. Rapidly decreasing levels together with a rising bilirubin level and prolongation of the prothrombin time portend a poor prognosis

347. Falsely lowered levels have been noted in azotemic patients

Gastroenterology
Answers

300. The answer is C. *(Braunwald, ed 11. pp 1260–1267.)* One of the causes of malabsorption, especially after surgery for peptic ulcer disease, is an overgrowth of bacteria in the small intestine. Unconjugated bile salts are usually not present in duodenal fluid, but they may be increased with bacterial overgrowth. Similarly, conjugated bile salts, which are normal in malabsorptive syndromes, may be decreased with bacterial overgrowth, especially when this is associated with ileal resection. The triolein absorption test correlates well with chemical stool fat and allows steatorrhea to be rapidly diagnosed. After the ingestion of ^{14}C triolein, the breath of the patient is examined to quantitate the excretion of $^{14}CO_2$ per hour. If greater than 3.5 percent of the dose is excreted per hour, the test is normal. In the presence of malabsorption or maldigestion associated with steatorrhea, excretion will be significantly reduced. The estimations of serum carotenes and serum vitamin A provide fairly satisfactory screening tests for malabsorption, but levels will be less than 100 IU/dl in both malabsorptive and maldigestive syndromes. Similarly, the quantitation of the amount of fat excreted in the stool is usually only of use in documenting the presence of steatorrhea. Values greater than 6 g in any 24-hour period are common in both pancreatic insufficiency and primary malabsorptive syndromes. The D-xylose absorption test is normal in pancreatic insufficiency, while a small intestinal mucosal biopsy will be normal with pancreatic insufficiency. Combining these tests with x-rays of the small intestines usually provides the physician with the means of arriving at a diagnosis for malabsorption.

301. The answer is A. *(Bozymski, Ann Intern Med 97:103–107, 1982.)* Patients with Barrett's esophagus typically present at age 50 to 70 after experiencing for several years symptoms of reflux esophagitis. Esophagoscopy with biopsy is the most widely used procedure for confirming the presence of this disorder, which is defined by the presence of columnar epithelium in the distal esophagus instead of the usual stratified squamous epithelium. Because pertechnetate selectively concentrates in ectopic gastric mucosa, some have suggested that a positive scan would eliminate the need for biopsy; however, because hiatal hernias are common in patients with Barrett's esophagus, the test is deemed unreliable. Complications associated with Barrett's esophagus are ulcer, stricture, dysplasia, and adenocarcinoma; in one series, 8.5 percent of patients developed adenocarcinoma of the esophagus. Because of this complication and its attendant poor prognosis, yearly endoscopic examinations with multiple biopsies are recommended. Management includes weight reduction, elevation of the head of the bed, antacids, and H_2-blockers. If symptoms persist, bethanechol or metoclopramide can be prescribed to raise sphincter pressure, hasten gastric emptying, and improve esophageal clearance.

302. The answer is D. *(Braunwald, ed 11. pp 1372–1376. Spiro, ed 3. pp 1013–1042.)* Although hyperlipemia and particularly hyperchylomicronemia may occur with acute pancreatitis, it is established that types I and V hyperlipidemias predispose to acute pancreatitis. Urinary clearance of amylase is markedly increased during acute pancreatitis, the amylase/creatinine clearance ratio usually being over 5; the reason for this is not entirely clear, although a defect in renal tubular reabsorption of amylase has been suggested. Pancreatic pseudocysts occur in approximately 10 percent of patients following acute pancreatitis. Although the management of pseudocysts is controversial, recent data indicate that internal drainage of a pseudocyst, before it has developed a fibrous capsule, has poor results. The danger associated with conservative therapy for pseudocysts is that of rupture. Therefore, indications for surgical intervention in a patient with a pseudocyst are (1) rapidly increasing size of pseudocyst, (2) development of an abscess, or (3) persistence of the pseudocyst for a period of 6 weeks. Although rupture of a pseudocyst increases mortality, the unsatisfactory results of immediate surgery suggest that observation for the first 6 weeks is in order provided that the complications mentioned above do not supervene. Hyperglycemia occurs in approximately 20 percent of affected patients, owing to an excess of released glucagon.

303. The answer is D. *(Braunwald, ed 11. pp 1315–1319.)* In all cases of alcoholic liver disease, γ-glutamyl transpeptidase is greatly elevated. This is a microsomal enzyme that is induced by alcohol. It may even be elevated in patients who consume large amounts of alcohol in the absence of liver disease. IgA frequently is increased in alcoholic liver injury and IgA:IgG sometimes is used to differentiate alcoholic from nonalcoholic liver disease. Smooth muscle antibody, however, is infrequently found in high titer in alcoholic liver disease and its presence suggests chronic active hepatitis. Prebetalipoproteins are increased in fatty liver; in cirrhosis, the prebeta band disappears almost completely. Frequently, all lipoproteins migrate as a single wide band. Hyperuricemia is caused by a high NADH:NAD ratio with hyperlactacidemia. This situation may lead to secondary hyperuricemia owing to decreased urine excretion of uric acid and may account for the common association of alcohol abuse and gout.

304. The answer is E. *(Braunwald, ed 11. p 1676. Spiro, ed 3. p 556.)* Polyarthritis occurs as a complication of jejunoileal bypass surgery presumably because of circulating immune complexes. Cholecystitis is a more frequent complication; it is probably due to the decreased bile acid pool that results from the malabsorption of bile acids. Fatty liver and even cirrhosis, often indistinguishable from that associated with chronic alcoholism, frequently develop in patients who have undergone jejunoileal bypass procedures. Although the histologic picture of chronic active hepatitis is not seen in these patients, Mallory bodies, centrilobular fibrosis, and neutrophilic infiltrates are noteworthy. Diarrhea, however, commonly occurs in this situation; it may be due to bile acid malabsorption, as well as to bacterial overgrowth.

305. The answer is D. *(Braunwald, ed 11. pp 1632–1635. Powell, Gastroenterology 78:374–381, 1980.)* The mainstay of therapy for idiopathic hemochromatosis continues to be routine phlebotomy. However, even in precirrhotic patients it will take between 18 and 24 months to reduce iron stores to acceptable levels. In older cirrhotic patients, the required duration of therapy may be longer. Usual treatment regimens include the weekly or biweekly removal of 500 ml of blood, a volume that contains 200 to 250 mg of iron. While this treatment initially may produce a mild anemia, stabilization of hemoglobin levels occurs within a few weeks and most affected patients tolerate the procedure well. In advanced stages of hemochromatosis and certainly in those patients who have developed cirrhosis, at least 25 g of iron must be removed. Thus, weekly phlebotomies for periods of up to 3 years are needed in some cases. While iron stores are being reduced to normal, routine phlebotomy is arranged to keep plasma iron levels at approximately 150 μg/100 ml. Constant checking for the possible reaccumulation of iron is necessary. This determination is made by carefully monitoring plasma iron levels and the percentage of saturation of transferrin with iron. Changes in these indices will precede any increases in serum ferritin concentration.

306. The answer is B. *(Braunwald, ed 11. p 1323.)* Recurrent cholestasis of pregnancy probably is due to an unusual sensitivity to estrogens. The condition occurs during the last trimester of pregnancy. Although it recurs with subsequent pregnancies, this form of cholestasis is a benign one.

307. The answer is C. *(Braunwald, ed 11. pp 1250–1252. Spiro, ed 3. p 310.)* Edema and swelling of the gastric and duodenal folds, as well as gastric hypersecretion with marked rugal hypertrophy, are characteristic of the Zollinger-Ellison syndrome. Although the syndrome may present with markedly atypical ulcers, the most common presenting manifestation is that of an uncomplicated duodenal ulcer. The best current definitive test for confirming the diagnosis of this syndrome is a direct assay of serum gastrin. Normal fasting levels range from 50 to 200 pg/ml, whereas in the Zollinger-Ellison syndrome, serum gastrin levels usually are greater than 1000 pg/ml.

308. The answer is E. *(Braunwald, ed 11. pp 1460–1461. Spiro, ed 3. pp 840–842.)* Ankylosing spondylitis has been observed in a significant number of patients with ulcerative colitis; the incidence of concurrence of these disorders is found to be as high as 30 percent in patients who have had ulcerative colitis for more than 10 years. Close relatives of patients with ulcerative colitis also have a higher incidence of ankylosing spondylitis than the normal population. Although sacroiliac disease with spondylitis also is fairly common in conjunction with ulcerative colitis, in most affected patients this lesion does not progress to florid ankylosis. Clubbing of the fingers also has been associated with ulcerative colitis, particularly if either the proximal part or large segments of the colon are involved. The association of ulcerative colitis with erythema multiforme is well described. Latex-negative arthritis, often involving large joints and often monarticular, is fairly common in association with ulcerative colitis. The joint symptoms frequently parallel the activity of the intestinal disease. Generally, joint disease is found more commonly in patients who have other evidence of extraintestinal manifestations of ulcerative colitis. Although the incidence of cholangiocarcinoma is increased in patients with ulcerative colitis, there is no increase in the incidence of hepatocellular carcinoma.

309. The answer is C. *(Mandell, ed 2. p 1667. Sleisenger, ed 3. pp 1318–1319.)* The differential diagnosis of proctitis is dominated by the infectious causes of enterocolitis. The clinical presentation typically includes mild-to-moderate rectal bleeding, a change in bowel habits, and tenesmus; systemic symptoms are unremarkable. On sigmoidoscopy, the rectal mucosa is shiny and hyperemic, bleeds easily on touching, and is sharply demarcated from the healthy bowel above. Biopsy shows changes typical of ulcerative colitis. Radiation proctitis, ulcerative proctitis, syphilis, *Campylobacter* infection, *Yersinia* infection, pseudomembranous colitis (antibiotic associated), and lymphogranuloma venereum should be considered, as well as the infections noted in the question (except giardiasis). In one series of proctitis in homosexual men, two or more pathogens were isolated from 11 percent of patients and in 42 percent no infectious cause was found.

310. The answer is B. *(Almy, N Engl J Med 302:324–329, 1980. Braunwald, ed 11. pp 1292, 1293. Spiro, ed 3. pp 745–746.)* Hemorrhage from diverticular disease is a common occurrence; it usually arises from uninflamed diverticula. Nevertheless, rectal bleeding must not be attributed to the presence of diverticulosis until other possible sources, including inflammatory bowel disease, angiodysplasia, carcinoma, and adenomata have been carefully excluded, usually by colonoscopy. If patients do bleed from diverticula, however, the outcome usually is good. Spontaneous cessation of bleeding is the rule and only in rare instances will conservative therapy fail to stop the bleeding. The characteristically mild course of the disease probably is attributable to the fact that small vessels (less than 1 mm in diameter) are generally involved. Diverticula usually form on the mesenteric location of the bowel, purportedly through sites in the muscle coats made vulnerable by the entrance of blood vessels.

311. The answer is B. *(Braunwald, ed 11. pp 1239–1253. Spiro, ed 3. pp 355–356.)* Although most benign gastric ulcers occur on the lesser curvature, some do occur on the greater curvature. The observation that an ulcer on the greater curvature is sharply punched out and is associated with radiating folds and Hampton's line favors the diagnosis of a benign ulcer. Biopsy at the time of gastroscopy is essential in the evaluation of a gastric ulcer. The presence of acid does not exclude the possibility of carcinoma; a gastric malignancy may be associated with high levels of acid. Most gastric ulcers heal in 6 weeks; an ulcer that has not healed by 8 weeks is an indication for surgery. Surgery in this circumstance is advisable both for fear of malignancy and because such ulcers tend to chronicity. Although gastric erosions and duodenal ulcers are more common in association with alcohol abuse, a history of alcoholism does not increase the likelihood of gastric ulceration.

312. The answer is D. *(Braunwald, ed 11. pp 1325–1336.)* Acute hepatitis A becomes increasingly less common with increasing age. Approximately 80 percent of urban adults over 50 years of age have already been exposed to hepatitis A and have IgG antibody to this antigen. It is unusual for acute hepatitis A to present with evidence of portal hypertension, like ascites, as early after exposure to possible sources of infection (clams) as is the case in the patient presented in the question. Moreover, the SGOT-SGPT ratio of greater than two virtually rules out any form of acute viral hepatitis. Acute hepatitis B is invariably associated with HBsAg and not with low titers of surface and core antibodies. The incubation period of non-A, non-B hepatitis following transfusion is 18 to 89 days. Although alpha methyldopa is an important cause of hypersensitivity hepatitis, the history of the patient presented makes drug-induced hepatitis unlikely. A large, firm liver with splenomegaly and ascites in a patient who drinks significantly, especially when the SGOT is significantly higher than the SGPT, makes alcoholic hepatitis the most likely diagnosis.

313. The answer is C. *(Braunwald, ed 11. pp 1321–1322.)* Gilbert's syndrome (unconjugated hyperbilirubinemia) is a benign condition in which there is defective hepatic uptake of unconjugated bilirubin. The prognosis for affected patients is excellent. Fasting causes a marked increase in the serum bilirubin level in this condition, whereas phenobarbital therapy may restore the level to normal.

314. The answer is D. *(Braunwald, ed 11. p 1297.)* With increasing human longevity, more and more vascular insufficiency affecting the small intestines is being encountered. A dull, but severe, aching pain usually comes on 15 minutes to 2 hours after the ingestion of food calls for an increased blood flow through the mesenteric vessels. If the patient does not eat he is less likely to experience the pain, and many subjects become quite cachexic as they become increasingly reluctant to eat. The pain will settle down spontaneously as the demand for blood flow decreases. The diagnosis can be made definitively only when a suspicious physician, having ruled out other abdominal causes, determines that mesenteric angiography is indicated. If the restriction of eating frequent small meals and the use of vasodilators do not relieve the condition, bypass surgery can occasionally be employed with success. Acute ischemia may present as a surgical emergency, and perforation of the bowel is a real possibility. Plain x-rays of the abdomen will reveal swollen bowel loops and their thickened walls. These changes look like those of regional enteritis, but the clinical pictures are entirely different. Patients with multisystem diseases that are caused by the deposition of immune complexes and the activation of complement may present with similar problems.

315. The answer is A. *(Braunwald, ed 11. pp 1341–1343.)* Alcoholic hepatitis, believed to be the precursor of cirrhosis in alcoholic liver disease, is diagnosed primarily on histologic examination. If affected patients continue to drink, a high percentage will develop cirrhosis. Approximately 25 percent of such patients who abstain from alcohol will recover over a period of 4 to 7 months.

316. The answer is D. *(Braunwald, ed 11. pp 1364–1366. Spiro, ed 3. pp 1117–1118.)* A stone in the common bile duct is visualized as a negative shadow on cholangiography. In addition, the common bile duct is dilated and a further obstruction is seen distal to the well-defined circular lesion. The patient discussed in the question offers a typical presentation of a common bile duct stone; carcinoma of the common bile duct, the pancreas, or the ampulla would be an unlikely diagnosis. A stone in the cystic duct does not cause an elevated bilirubin level of the order of 10 mg/100 ml and the filling defect in the common bile duct is further evidence against such a diagnosis.

317. The answer is A. *(Braunwald, ed 11. pp 406–410. Force, Surgery 88:17, 1980.)* It has been estimated that between 30 and 50 percent of all patients in major hospitals where intensive medical care is delivered are significantly malnourished. Recent advances in our ability to deliver adequate nutrition parenterally are making it possible for this situation to be significantly improved. Patients who are malnourished, especially those who have recently lost a considerable amount of weight, are more susceptible to infection and have poorer wound healing, and operative mortality is higher. Any patient with 10 percent or greater loss of body weight should be reviewed to determine if nutritional support is required. For a number of patients, this may be accomplished by enteral tube feedings, but the real advances have come from the better techniques that allow sophisticated preparations to be delivered through either a peripheral or central vein. All essential nutrients and 3000 kcal can be supplied to patients via an infusion into the superior vena cava, providing the patient can tolerate 2 to 3 L of intravenous fluids daily. Commonly the solutions infused consist of 50% dextrose and an equal volume of an 8.5% amino acid solution. On such a regimen, patients should be weighed daily and have their fluid and nutritional balance charts kept meticulously. Urine and glucose should be monitored at least every 6 hours, more frequently in diabetic subjects. Although in some diabetic subjects the presence of glucose in the urine does not correlate with hyperglycemia, for most diabetics and nondiabetic subjects glycosuria is likely to be associated with hypoglycemia and severe osmotic diuresis that may lead to dehydration. If 7000 kcal above metabolic demands can be supplied on a weekly basis, patients are likely to gain 1 kg/week in body weight, which has been determined to be satisfactory. Considerable advances in our knowledge about methods for infusing fat emulsions have improved parenteral nutrition. Fat provides more energy per unit weight than does either carbohydrate or protein. The body can synthesize most long chain fatty acids, but linoleic and linolenic acids must be supplied. The goal of parenteral nutrition is to supply 4 to 10 percent of the daily caloric requirement as essential fatty acids. Two to three 500-ml bottles of a 10% fat emulsion per week will usually be adequate for this purpose.

318. The answer is D. *(Braunwald, ed 11. p 1270. Sleisenger, ed 3. pp 921–922.)* Scleroderma frequently involves the small intestine, resulting in dilated bowel loops and intestinal stasis. Bacterial overgrowth commonly accompanies the stasis. The malabsorption of scleroderma often can be effectively treated with broad-spectrum antibiotics.

319. The answer is A. *(Braunwald, ed 11. p 1354. Waldman, JAMA 247:308–309, 1982.)* Although commonly thought of as a complication of viral illnesses in children, Reye's syndrome has recently been described in both young and middle-aged adults. The cause of this condition is unclear, but it appears to develop when certain viral infections and salicylates combine to produce severe acute liver damage. So serious is the condition that in children it is recommended that salicylates not be given when a diagnosis of influenza or chickenpox is suspected. The clinical story detailed in this question is typical for the syndrome. Prothrombin time is often prolonged, which may make it difficult to get a liver biopsy early in the illness; but where it can be obtained, microvesicular steatosis with little or no inflammation will be observed. Clues to the disturbance have been provided by careful electromicroscopic examination of affected liver where it can readily be seen that the mitochondria are severely damaged. Therapy consists of treatment of the liver failure and seizure activity. Steroids are often used to lower increased intracranial pressure. Nearly 25 percent of patients with this syndrome will die despite supportive efforts. Severe renal and hepatic damage can be caused by the wild mushroom *Amanita phalloides*. Even small amounts will have a direct toxic effect on liver cells, producing irreversible hepatic necrosis. The mortality is high. Although leptospirosis can affect the liver and produce a meningitis, the most common findings are bradycardia, muscle tenderness, and a stiff neck. A nonpurulent conjunctivitis may supply a valuable clue. Hepatomegaly is uncommon. Encephalitis can be caused by eastern and western equine encephalitis viruses, which are togaviruses, but the liver is usually not involved. Disseminated cytomegalovirus infection can affect the liver and the brain but only occurs in immunocompromised adults.

320. The answer is B (1, 3). *(Braunwald, ed 11. p 1367.)* Sclerosing cholangitis is an uncommon condition that is characterized by a progressively obliterative process of the bile ducts, both extra- and intrahepatic. Many of these patients have ulcerative colitis, although sclerosing cholangitis may be seen secondary to long-standing choledocholithiasis. Clinical presentation is frequently as seen in the patient presented, with jaundice, pruritus, and right upper quadrant pain; laboratory studies reveal negative serologic tests. Diagnosis is confirmed by the typical features seen on cholangiography—thickened bile duct walls with beaded lumina. Therapeutic measures have been disappointing and prognosis is generally poor.

321. The answer is E (all). *(Braunwald, ed 11. p 1274.)* Deficiency of mucosal lactase is associated with symptoms of intolerance upon ingestion of lactose: abdominal cramps, bloating, and diarrhea are typical of this condition. The symptoms are due to the osmotic effect of unabsorbed lactose, which leads to shifts of fluid into the intestinal lumen. In addition, colonic bacteria ferment lactose to lactic acid and short-chain fatty acids, which leads to a decrease in stool pH. The diagnosis of lactase deficiency can be made by administering an oral dose of lactose and obtaining serial measurements of blood glucose; lactose intolerance is diagnosed if intestinal symptoms occur and the blood glucose increases less than 20 mg/dl above the fasting level. Because false positive and false negative tests occur in 20 percent of normal persons, measurement of breath hydrogen after ingestion of 50 g lactose, a more sensitive and specific test, is preferred. Gastrointestinal disease in which lactase deficiency is often seen include tropical and nontropical sprue, ulcerative colitis, regional enteritis, giardiasis, viral and bacterial infections of the intestine, cystic fibrosis, and abetalipoproteinemia.

322. The answer is A (1, 2, 3). *(Mandell, ed 2. pp 791–795.)* Granulomatous hepatitis is a common clinical entity and may be found in up to 10 percent of liver biopsy specimens. It most often represents a systemic granulomatous disease and rarely is it a process isolated to the liver. Pathogenetically, it involves the transformation of monocyte macrophages into epithelioid cells either by chronic antigen exposure, circulating immune complexes, or by mediators released by lymphocytes. Hepatic granulomata are nodular infiltrates of these epithelioid cells. The causes of granulomatous hepatitis are many and are broadly classified into infectious and noninfectious causes. The most common infectious causes include tuberculosis, histoplasmosis, cytomegalovirus, infectious mononucleosis, schistosomiasis, and syphilis. The noninfectious causes include sarcoidosis, erythema nodosum, primary biliary cirrhosis, Hodgkin's disease, and allergic granulomatosis. In one series, 37 of 72 cases remained undiagnosed. Fever is a common finding. Laboratory abnormalities are nonspecific and liver function tests may, in fact, be normal.

323. The answer is B (1, 3). *(Braunwald, ed 11. pp 484, 1376.)* Pancreatic abscesses are a serious complication of pancreatitis and occur in 1 to 4 percent of cases. They are caused by secondary infection of necrotic tissue, where they usually form multiple foci. They are commonly polymicrobial; anaerobic organisms, gram-negative aerobic bacilli, enterococci, and staphylococci are common pathogens. In patients receiving hyperalimentation, *Candida* may be a causative organism, as well. Pancreatic abscesses occur 2 or more weeks after presentation, rarely sooner, and should be suspected in any patient who suddenly deteriorates after initial clinical improvement. Ultrasound and computerized tomography are useful in establishing the diagnosis. Therapy includes broad-spectrum antibiotic coverage and surgical drainage. Mortality approaches 40 percent even with surgical drainage, and recurrent abscesses are common.

324. The answer is D (4). *(Spiro, ed 3. pp 69–82.)* Achalasia is an esophageal disorder characterized by an elevated lower esophageal sphincter pressure with reduced relaxation after swallowing and aperistalsis of the body of the esophagus. It most commonly is a disease of adults and characteristically presents as an intermittent, painless dysphagia with both solids and liquids. Belching and vomiting occur rarely and weight loss may become quite significant with time. Diagnosis is made on barium swallow, which will usually show a dilated esophagus, a narrow, conical lower segment, and very little esophageal motility. In equivocal cases, manometry will confirm the diagnosis. Medical therapy of achalasia includes nitrates, calcium channel blockers, beta blockers, and bougienage. Surgical treatment in refractory cases consists of a single myotomy of the esophagus and has a success rate approximating 85 percent, about the same as medical therapy. Prognosis is generally good, although the incidence of esophageal carcinoma hovers around 5 percent.

325. The answer is C (2, 4). *(Braunwald, ed 11. p 1346.)* The Budd-Chiari syndrome is associated with myeloproliferative disease, tumors, use of oral contraceptives, and pregnancy. The existence of a fibrous diaphragm across the upper vena cava, which is one of the causes of the syndrome, is important to identify because it is treatable. Most affected patients present with a painful, tender liver and severe ascites resistant to therapy. Portal hypertension occurs late in the course of the illness. Liver scanning with technetium (^{99m}Tc) shows central uptake of colloid in the caudate lobe, together with reduced uptake in the right lobe. This pattern of uptake is thought to be due to the fact that the caudate lobe often drains directly into the inferior vena cava. Although therapy often is unsuccessful, side-to-side shunt has proved useful in a number of cases.

326. The answer is B (1, 3). *(Braunwald, ed 11. pp 1344–1345.)* Approximately 90 percent of primary biliary cirrhosis cases occur in women. The usually insidious onset is characterized by pruritus and fatigue. Jaundice is a relatively late finding. There is no effective treatment for this disease; corticosteroids have not been shown to be of use. Although penicillamine has been shown to decrease the amount of copper in the liver, there has been no success with this drug in the long-term treatment of primary biliary cirrhosis, nor is there evidence that penicillamine effectively reduces bile duct injury. Gallstones occur with greater frequency in primary biliary cirrhosis than in other forms of cirrhosis.

327. The answer is A (1, 2, 3). *(Braunwald, ed 11. pp 1333, 1338–1340.)* In chronic active hepatitis, HBeAg correlates with the number of Dane particles and the infectiousness of the serum. It does not correlate well with the degree of activity of the liver disease, but is not uncommon in association with chronic active hepatitis. Anti-HBc is almost invariably present when HBsAg is detected in serum, whereas anti-HBs is not usually found by radioimmunoassay in the presence of HBsAg. Anti-HA (IgG) is found in up to 80 percent of affected adults over 50 years of age.

328. The answer is B (1, 3). *(Braunwald, ed 11. pp 1325–1328, 1330.)* Non-A, non-B hepatitis currently accounts for approximately 20 percent of sporadic hepatitis. There have been a number of reports in which non-A, non-B hepatitis has occurred without percutaneous exposure. Anicteric hepatitis is two to three times more common than icteric hepatitis. Current studies have not conclusively shown that immune serum globulin prevents the total incidence of non-A, non-B hepatitis if given after exposure. The only study in which a protective effect of gamma globulin was shown was one in which the gamma globulin was given prophylactically to patients receiving multiple transfusions during open heart surgery. Although the propensity to develop chronic hepatitis after non-A, non-B hepatitis is as great as, if not greater than, that following hepatitis B, the course of the disease appears to be milder than hepatitis B. According to one recent study, the course of non-A, non-B hepatitis appeared to decrease in severity with time.

329. The answer is C (2, 4). *(Braunwald, ed 11. pp 1252–1253. Gottlieb, Am J Gastroenterol 81:227–238, 1986.)* Gastrointestinal erosions and ulcerations are common complications in patients admitted to an intensive care unit, with an incidence ranging from 70 to 100 percent. They are superficial lesions, frequently multiple, and have a tendency to occur in the fundic mucosa in contrast to other peptic ulcers, which typically occur in the gastric antrum or duodenum. They develop approximately 24 hours after the acute insult and, while their most frequent presentation is painless bleeding, only 20 percent of stress ulcers do hemorrhage. All stress ulcers are associated with a higher mortality, although associated bleeding worsens the prognosis even further. While their pathogenesis is disputed, lowering gastric pH seems to be preventive. The frequency of stress ulcers is reduced by either antacids or cimetidine, each having its advocates in particular clinical situations.

330. The answer is D (4). *(Spiro, ed 3. pp 623–629.)* Whipple's disease is a cause of steatorrhea characterized by the finding of many PAS-positive macrophages in the lamina propria of the small intestine. It is typically associated with low-grade fever, nondeforming polyarthritis, abdominal pain, peripheral lymphadenopathy, diarrhea, and a diffuse skin pigmentation that, unlike Addison's disease, spares the buccal mucosa. Neurologic abnormalities include memory loss, confusion, somnolence, and polydipsia; CNS involvement may precede the gastrointestinal manifestations of this disease. Antibiotic therapy with tetracycline for 2 months results in a long remission. Steroids may be used in conjunction with antibiotics to hasten the reversal of symptoms.

331. The answer is D (4). *(Berk, ed 4. pp 3222–3235.)* Wilson's disease is characterized by an abnormality of hepatic copper excretion and demonstrates autosomal recessive inheritance. Most patients present in their teens, although older patients are not uncommon. Pathogenetically, the accumulated copper inhibits ceruloplasmin synthesis, and levels within hepatocytes rise. Once the liver's capacity to store copper is exceeded, copper is released into the bloodstream and is taken up by extrahepatic tissues. Wilson's disease may present with several hepatic manifestations ranging from a fulminant deterioration, to a picture similar to that of chronic active hepatitis, to a self-limiting form of acute hepatitis. The neuropsychiatric abnormality typically manifests as a motor dysfunction and a myriad of psychiatric disturbances. A Coombs-negative hemolytic anemia and amenorrhea are common manifestations, as well. Laboratory abnormalities include an elevated serum copper, a low ceruloplasmin level (although any parenchymal liver disease may result in low levels of the protein), and a greater than 50 μg per day urinary excretion rate of copper. Treatment involves lifelong therapy with penicillamine.

332. The answer is A (1, 2, 3). *(Sleisenger, ed 3. pp 49–51, 1023–1038.)* An overgrowth of bacteria in the small intestine may be caused by any abnormality that results in local stasis or impaired gastric acid secretion. The causes of this entity are many and include enteroenterostomy, Crohn's disease, diverticula, scleroderma, diabetic autonomic dysfunction, and achlorhydria. The overgrowth is polymicrobial and resembles the bacterial flora of feces. Several species of bacteria bind cobalamin and thereby produce intrinsic factor–resistant B_{12} deficiency. Conversely, bacteria produce folate, which is available for absorption. Fat malabsorption is secondary to altered bile salt metabolism while direct mucosal damage, manifest as a moderate blunting of villi, is probably responsible for protein and polysaccharide malabsorption. Antibiotic therapy with tetracycline, metronidazole, clindamycin, or chloramphenicol produces, in most patients, freedom from symptoms for months after just 7 to 10 days of therapy.

333–337. The answers are: 333-A, 334-B, 335-A, 336-A, 337-A. *(Braunwald, ed 11. pp 1338–1340.)* Chronic hepatitis refers to a combination of hepatic necrosis and inflammation lasting for more than 6 months. Chronic persistent hepatitis is the result of infection with hepatitis B virus and non-A, non-B hepatitis virus. Progression to cirrhosis is very rare and hepatic failure is not seen. In 70 percent of patients, the onset is like that of acute hepatitis; patients may complain of anorexia, fatigue, nausea, and vomiting. Biopsy reveals mononuclear cell infiltration of the portal areas and only rarely is there erosion of the limiting plate; the lobular architecture is preserved. Because these patients generally do not develop cirrhosis, no specific therapy is required.

Chronic active hepatitis is characterized by continuing hepatic necrosis, active inflammation, and fibrosis. Liver biopsy reveals the following: a mononuclear and plasma cell infiltration of the portal zones extending into the liver lobule, erosion of the limiting plate, connective tissue septa extending from the portal zones into the lobule, and evidence of hepatic generation. Cirrhosis can be demonstrated in 20 to 50 percent of patients. Etiologic agents include hepatitis B virus; non-A, non-B hepatitis virus; and drugs such as methyldopa, isoniazid, and nitrofurantoin. Associated diseases include diabetes mellitus, thyroiditis, ulcerative colitis, Coombs-positive hemolytic anemia, proliferative glomerulonephritis, and Sjögren's syndrome. In two-thirds of patients, the disease has an insidious onset with fatigue, jaundice, malaise, anorexia, and fever being common symptoms. Extrahepatic involvement—such as abdominal pain, arthralgias or arthritis, pericarditis, and sicca syndrome—is common. Corticosteroid therapy is the treatment of choice in symptomatic HBsAg-negative and severe chronic hepatitis; the dosage of steroid may be lowered with the concomitant administration of azathioprine, but this latter agent is not effective alone. Corticosteroids have no effect on the natural course of HBsAg-positive chronic active hepatitis.

338–342. The answers are: 338-A, 339-B, 340-B, 341-C, 342-D. *(Braunwald, ed 11. p 1299. Case Records of the MGH Case 2-1988, N Engl J Med 318:100–109, 1988.)* The familial polyposis syndromes are all inherited in an autosomal dominant pattern and may be divided into adenomatous and hamartomatous forms of polyposis based on the histologic features of the lesions.

Both familial polyposis coli and Gardner's syndrome are adenomatous polyposis syndromes characterized by numerous polyps involving the entire colon. In familial polyposis coli, the polyps appear in childhood and adolescence and may cause bleeding and diarrhea. Because cancer of the colon is inevitable by age 40, proctocolectomy is advised at the time of diagnosis. In addition, it is imperative to screen family members for presence of the disease.

Gardner's syndrome involves adenomatous polyps of the colon and duodenum, benign soft tissue tumors, and osteomas, particularly of the jaw and skull. Congenital hypertrophy of retinal pigment epithelium, diagnosed on fundoscopic examination, is also described and may precede the other characteristics of the syndrome. Because the risk of carcinoma is the same as found in familial polyposis coli, colectomy is also recommended.

The hamartomatous forms of polyposis include the Peutz-Jeghers syndrome, Cowden's disease, neurofibromatosis, and juvenile polyposis. The Peutz-Jeghers syndrome is characterized by multiple hamartomatous polyps of the entire gastrointestinal tract associated with melanotic spots of the lips, skin, and buccal mucosa; patients often present with obstruction or intussusception due to the mass effect of the polyp. Cowden's syndrome involves multiple hamartomas in diverse tissues associated with adenomas or carcinomas of multiple tissue types. Juvenile polyposis involves histologically varied polyps that may occur anywhere in the gastrointestinal tract. Clinical presentation includes rectal bleeding, diarrhea, rectal prolapse of a polyp, intussusception, and abdominal pain.

343–347. The answers are: 343-D, 344-C, 345-D, 346-C, 347-D. *(Chopra, Am J Med 79:221–230, 1985.)* Both SGPT, a cytosolic enzyme also called alanine aminotransferase, and SGOT, a mitochondrial enzyme sometimes referred to as aspartate aminotransferase, are commonly used indicators of liver dysfunction. While SGPT is found primarily in the liver, SGOT is present in many tissues, including heart, skeletal muscle, kidney, and brain, and is therefore a less specific indicator of liver disease.

The highest elevations of the transaminases are encountered in conditions causing extensive hepatic necrosis such as acute viral hepatitis, toxin-induced liver damage, and ischemic hepatitis; however, the absolute levels of these enzymes correlate poorly with the extent of liver cell necrosis and prognosis. Lesser elevations are found in both diffuse and chronic liver diseases such as cirrhosis, chronic active hepatitis, and hepatic metastases; in uncomplicated extrahepatic obstruction, levels are generally less than 1000 IU. In severe alcoholic hepatitis, only modest increases in the transaminases are found and the SGOT/SGPT ratio may be greater than 2. While assays of both SGOT and SGPT are indicators of hepatocellular damage, rapidly decreasing levels in conjunction with rising levels of bilirubin and a prolongation of the prothrombin time together portend a poor prognosis as they indicate extensive damage of the liver. Of note, uremia may lead to spuriously low levels of aminotransferase.

Diseases of the Urinary Tract

DIRECTIONS: Each question below contains five suggested responses. Select the **one best** response to each question.

348. All the following measures are advisable for the patient suffering from nephrolithiasis caused by calcium oxalate stones EXCEPT that

(A) to dilute urine metabolites patients should drink 2 to 3 L of fluid per day and monitor their urine's specific gravity to maintain it in the range of 1.005 to 1.010
(B) patients should avoid drinking tea, chocolate, and other fluids that contain oxalates
(C) thiazide diuretics should be avoided as they can aggravate stone inflammation by causing both dehydration and hypercalcemia
(D) allopurinol can reduce the formation of calcium oxalate stones in patients with hyperuricosuria
(E) orthophosphate therapy, though helpful, is frequently poorly tolerated because of the severe diarrhea it causes

349. Which of the following conditions may be responsible for a metabolic alkalosis associated with a urinary chloride concentration less than 20 mEq/L?

(A) Cushing's syndrome
(B) Primary aldosteronism
(C) Bartter's syndrome
(D) Diuretic abuse
(E) Vomiting

350. A characteristic of poststreptococcal glomerulonephritis is that it

(A) follows infection by group B, alpha-hemolytic streptococci
(B) is prevented by prompt treatment of the inciting infection
(C) may occur at the same time as the infection
(D) is associated with a decline in the C3 component of complement
(E) rarely evolves into chronic progressive glomerulonephritis in sporadic adult cases

351. The most common renal neo-plasm is a hypernephroma. This tumor is associated with all the following conditions EXCEPT

(A) liver function abnormalities in the absence of hepatic metastases
(B) pancytopenia in the absence of marrow metastases
(C) anemia
(D) thrombocytosis
(E) eosinophilia

DIRECTIONS: Each question below contains four suggested responses of which **one or more** is correct. Select

A	if	**1, 2, and 3**	are correct
B	if	**1 and 3**	are correct
C	if	**2 and 4**	are correct
D	if	**4**	is correct
E	if	**1, 2, 3, and 4**	are correct

352. True statements concerning renal disease associated with multiple myeloma include which of the following?

(1) The Fanconi syndrome occurs mainly in patients who excrete kappa light chains

(2) Plasmapheresis is more effective than peritoneal dialysis in removing light chains

(3) The major cause of renal failure is the excretion of light chains

(4) Hematuria is commonly the earliest manifestation of renal disease

353. True statements concerning preeclampsia include which of the following?

(1) Red blood cells and cellular casts are frequently found in the urinary sediment

(2) Proteinuria may precede the hypertension and edema

(3) A blood urea nitrogen (BUN) of 20 mg/dl is usually indicative of normal renal function

(4) Proteinuria and hypertension may persist for as long as 6 months after emptying the uterus

354. True statements concerning hyperkalemic periodic paralysis include

(1) it is transmitted in autosomal dominant fashion

(2) patients typically have compromised renal function

(3) exposure to cold may precipitate attacks

(4) thiazide diuretics are contraindicated in patients with this disorder

355. True statements concerning peritoneal dialysis include which of the following?

(1) In contrast to hemodialysis, clearance rates of small molecules are not blood-flow dependent

(2) In diabetic patients receiving peritoneal dialysis, good control of blood glucose levels can be achieved by adding insulin to the dialysis solution

(3) During peritonitis, the ultrafiltration rate falls

(4) Lactate and acetate in peritoneal dialysis solutions are equally effective in correcting uremic acidosis during routine dialysis

356. The renal effects of hypokalemia include which of the following?

(1) Urine concentrating ability decreases

(2) Renal parenchymal production of ammonia increases

(3) Phosphate excretion increases

(4) A ballooning of glomerular endothelial cells occurs

357. Epididymitis is correctly represented by which of the following statements?

(1) It may be differentiated from torsion of the testicle by urethral smear

(2) It may require treatment of sexual partners

(3) Infection due to coliform bacteria implies an underlying structural or functional genitourinary abnormality

(4) Dysuria is common

358. The nephrotic syndrome is associated with

(1) low T_4 and enhanced resin T_3 uptake

(2) unilateral and bilateral renal vein thrombosis

(3) Goodpasture's syndrome

(4) Wilms's tumor

359. Sickle cell nephropathy is associated with

(1) gross, painless hematuria

(2) failure of urinary concentration

(3) papillary necrosis

(4) dialysis in its last stages

360. Correct statements concerning membranous glomerulopathy include which of the following?

(1) Rare cases have recurred in renal transplants

(2) The most common associated tumor is of the breast

(3) Children have a better prognosis than adults

(4) Renal vein thrombosis is a rare complication

361. True statements concerning renal vein thrombosis include which of the following?

(1) In children it may be secondary to dehydration

(2) It occurs in conjunction with hypernephromas

(3) Its initial symptoms are hematuria and proteinuria

(4) It is rarely bilateral

362. Prostatectomy may cause which of the following complications?

(1) Urinary incontinence

(2) Retrograde ejaculation

(3) Urethral stricture formation

(4) Epididymitis

363. Adult polycystic kidney disease is characterized by

(1) progressive renal insufficiency
(2) large multicystic kidneys
(3) increased incidence of cerebral aneurysms
(4) autosomal recessive inheritance

364. Carcinoma of the urinary bladder is characterized by which of the following statements?

(1) It is usually an adenocarcinoma
(2) It has a higher-than-average incidence in those who smoke cigarettes heavily
(3) It is frequently a metastatic lesion
(4) It commonly presents with painless hematuria

DIRECTIONS: Each group of questions below consists of four lettered headings followed by a set of numbered items. For each numbered item select

A	if the item is associated with	(A) **only**
B	if the item is associated with	(B) **only**
C	if the item is associated with	**both** (A) and (B)
D	if the item is associated with	**neither** (A) nor (B)

Each lettered heading may be used **once, more than once, or not at all.**

Questions 365–368

(A) Medullary sponge kidney
(B) Medullary cystic kidney disease
(C) Both
(D) Neither

365. End-stage renal failure invariably results

366. Patients typically present with nocturia

367. Urinalysis is characteristically normal

368. Distal renal tubule acidosis results

Questions 369–373

(A) Polyarteritis nodosa
(B) Churg-Strauss disease
(C) Both
(D) Neither

369. Vasculitis involves small- and medium-sized muscular arteries, capillaries, veins, and venules

370. Lung involvement is predominant

371. Renal failure occurs in less than 10 percent of patients

372. Hypertension is common

373. Complement levels are normal

Diseases of
the Urinary Tract
Answers

348. **The answer is C.** *(Braunwald, ed 11. pp 1211–1215. Peacock, Drugs 20:225, 1980.)* Sixty-five percent of all renal stones are composed of calcium oxalate. Decreased levels of calcium in the blood are usually associated with increased urinary calcium. Hyperuricosuria is present in 25 percent of patients who have calcium oxalate stones and appears to contribute to the stones' formation. Hyperoxaluria, although uncommon, occurs following excessive intestinal absorption of ingested oxalate and can predispose to the formation of stones in the urinary tract. Although there is no consensus about the ideal management of patients troubled by calcium oxalate stones, a number of measures of importance have become clear. Patients should certainly be encouraged to keep their urine dilute, and there is evidence that the avoidance of fluids containing oxalate, such as tea and chocolate and some fruit juices, is of benefit. Thiazide diuretics are certainly not contraindicated in the management of calcium oxalate stones, and many investigators feel they are of considerable therapeutic benefit. Stone enlargement ceased in 90 percent of patients who took hydrochlorthiazide twice daily on a regular basis in one study. In patients who have calcium oxalate stones and hyperuricosuria, the administration of allopurinol to reduce uric acid excretion to less than 650 mg/day reduced the rate of calcium oxalate stones in patients by 90 percent in one study. The combination of allopurinol and a thiazide diuretic is advocated by many specialists in this area. Orthophosphate therapy does tend to produce diarrhea and dyspepsia, but excellent results have been obtained in many patients taking these reagents. Phosphates appear to increase the excretion into the urine of substances that block crystal formation.

349. **The answer is E.** *(Maxwell, ed 4. pp 702–706.)* The mean concentrations of the components of gastric fluid are as follows: sodium 20 mEq/L, potassium 10 mEq/L, chloride 120 mEq/L, and hydrogen ion 90 mEq/L. With vomiting, each milliequivalent of hydrochloric acid lost from the stomach reciprocates as 1 mEq of bicarbonate added to the extracellular fluid. As the plasma bicarbonate rises, the reabsorptive capacity of the proximal tubule is exceeded and bicarbonate is delivered to the distal tubule as sodium bicarbonate; here some of the sodium is exchanged for potassium. Owing to the loss of gastric juice, the urinary chloride concentration is low. As arterial blood volume falls, however, proximal bicarbonate absorption is increased and aldosterone secretion is increased. Then, as potassium stores fall, aldosterone secretion falls as well, while proximal bicarbonate absorption remains high because of volume contraction and hypokalemia. Owing to the various stages involved in protracted vomiting, urinary chloride concentration, not the sodium concentration, is an accurate marker of the volume status of the patient. Indeed, a urinary chloride concentration greater than 40 mEq/L indicates that sufficient salt replacement has been given.

350. The answer is D. *(Braunwald, ed 11. pp 1174–1175.)* Poststreptococcal glomerulonephritis is caused by a preceding infection of the throat or skin by nephritogenic strains of group A, beta-hemolytic streptococci. A latent period of 6 days to 2 weeks always exists between the infection and the nephritis; indeed, absence of a latent period implies an exacerbation of a previously unrecognized renal lesion. The diagnosis of poststreptococcal glomerulonephritis rests on the demonstration of antibodies to any of the streptococcal exoenzymes, presence of nephritogenic streptococci, or a transient decline in the C3 component of complement. Unlike rheumatic fever, the nephritis is not prevented by treatment of the antecedent infection. Generally, though, prognosis is good except in sporadic cases of poststreptococcal glomerulonephritis in adults, which may evolve into chronic progressive glomerulonephritis in as many as 40 percent of cases.

351. The answer is B. *(Braunwald, ed 11. p 1218.)* Common systemic symptoms and sequelae of hypernephroma include (1) fatigability, (2) weight loss, (3) cachexia, (4) fever, and (5) anemia. Erythrocytosis occurs in about 5 percent of affected patients; it is probably associated with erythropoietin production. Eosinophilia, leukemoid reaction, thrombocytosis, and elevated erythrocyte sedimentation rate are also observed. Hematuria, usually microscopic, is commonly present. Patients sometimes demonstrate reversible liver function disturbances. These disturbances occur even when hepatic metastases are not present. Pancytopenia in the absence of bone marrow involvement, however, is not a characteristic feature of hypernephroma.

352. The answer is A (1, 2, 3). *(Williams, ed 3. pp 1083–1084, 1096.)* Multiple myeloma is a plasma cell neoplasm whose main features are bone marrow dysfunction, renal failure, bone destruction, and hypercalcemia. Renal disease is a common complication of myeloma caused predominantly by damage of renal tubule cells by light chains. The nephrotoxicity of light chains, however, is variable. Renal insufficiency is more common in patients who excrete lambda chains, while the Fanconi syndrome occurs mainly in patients excreting kappa light chains. Therapy for patients who develop renal failure in the face of excessive excretion of light chains involves chemotherapy and plasmapheresis, which is ten times more effective than peritoneal dialysis in removing light chains. The presence of uremia in multiple myeloma is a poor prognostic sign; patients with a blood urea nitrogen concentration of greater than 80 have only a 2-month survival.

353. The answer is C (2, 4). *(Braunwald, ed 11. p 1204.)* Preeclampsia is characterized by hypertension, edema, and proteinuria during gestation or within 7 days of delivery. With severe hypertension, convulsions and coma may occur and the disorder is termed eclampsia. The onset may be insidious or abrupt with headache, visual disturbances, epigastric distress, and apprehension. Hypertension, defined as pressure exceeding 125/75, and edema generally appear together, with proteinuria usually following but occasionally preceding the diad. The urine may contain up to 10 g protein per 24 hours as well as granular and hyalin casts. Treatment ranges from simple bed rest and mild sedation to termination of pregnancy. After emptying the uterus, the hypertension and proteinuria usually resolve in 6 weeks but may persist for 6 months.

354. The answer is B (1, 3). *(Maxwell, p 569.)* Hyperkalemic periodic paralysis is a disorder characterized by transient attacks of paralysis and hyperkalemia in persons with normal renal, adrenal, and pancreatic function; it is transmitted in autosomal dominant fashion. During attacks, the muscle concentration of potassium falls, while the plasma concentration rises; the resultant alteration in the ratio of intracellular to extracellular potassium leads to paralysis. Exercise, exposure to cold, and potassium administration precipitate attacks, while a high-carbohydrate diet, thiazide diuretics, and albuterol (salbutamol in Canada and Europe) decrease the frequency and severity of the attacks.

355. The answer is E (all). *(Maxwell, pp 1077–1085.)* The peritoneum is analogous to a dialyzing membrane; indeed, while only a fraction of the peritoneum is functionally available for dialysis transport, the peritoneum is more permeable than hemodialysis membranes to solutes in the middle range of molecular weights. In further contradistinction to hemodialysis, clearance rates of small molecules such as urea are not limited by solute delivery, or blood-flow rate, but rather by a diffusion barrier. Dialyzable solutes move between blood and the intraperitoneal dialysis solution along individual concentration gradients; ultrafiltration across the peritoneal membrane is accomplished by osmotic gradient differences created by the addition of dextrose to the dialysate. Peritoneal dialysis solutions contain either acetate or lactate in concentrations ranging from 35 to 45 mEq/L to correct uremic acidosis as both are metabolized in the body to bicarbonate. Other components of premixed dialysis solutions are sodium, calcium, magnesium, and chloride; insulin may be added to maintain good glucose control in diabetic patients on chronic peritoneal dialysis. Advantages of peritoneal dialysis are avoidance of heparinization and vascular surgery, and a slower clearance rate in patients with cardiovascular instability. Disadvantages include peritonitis, protein loss, hypertriglyceridemia, hypercholesterolemia, and inguinal and abdominal hernias.

356. The answer is A (1, 2, 3). *(Braunwald, ed 11. pp 205–207.)* Regardless of cause, renal dysfunction seen in hypokalemia remains constant. Decreased urine concentration, increased ammonia production, and increased phosphate excretion are manifest clinically as polyuria, polydipsia, nocturia, muscle weakness, and a decrease in maximum urinary acidification. Histologically, hypokalemic nephropathy is characterized by vacuolization of renal tubule cells with sparing of glomeruli and blood vessels. These changes are reversed with potassium repletion, although it is debated whether interstitial scarring may result from prolonged or recurrent potassium depletion.

357. The answer is A (1, 2, 3). *(Holmes, pp 650–661.)* Epididymitis, a common infection, is almost always unilateral and presents typically with severe scrotal pain of relatively acute onset and fever; symptoms of dysuria are surprisingly infrequent. The bacteriology of this condition differs among various age groups. In prepubertal children and men over 35, coliform bacteria and *Pseudomonas aeruginosa* are the usual pathogens. The causes are often uncorrected congenital anomalies in children and the occurrence of acquired structural or functional disorders in older men. In men under 35, *Chlamydia trachomatis* and *Neisseria gonorrhoeae* are the most common pathogens and typically occur in patients who have multiple sexual partners. Treatment in this group requires treatment of sexual partners, as well. Diagnosis involves a urethral smear that should be sent for culture and Gram stained. While epididymitis does not always imply concurrent urethritis, the presence of urethral leukocytes effectively rules out torsion of the testis.

358. The answer is E (all). *(Braunwald, ed 11. pp 1176–1182.)* The nephrotic syndrome is characterized by proteinuria in excess of 3.5 g per 1.73 m^2 per day, hypoalbuminemia, hyperlipidemia, and edema. The proteinuria involves plasma proteins and albumin. Indeed, urinary losses of transferrin, thyroxine-binding globulin (which results in low T_4 and enhanced resin T_3 uptake), and vitamin D–binding protein may give rise to various deficiency states; loss of antithrombin III may be responsible for a hypercoagulable state and resultant renal vein thrombosis. Causes of the nephrotic syndrome include primary glomerular diseases and those secondary to infections, neoplasms (e.g., Wilms's tumor), medications, metabolic diseases, connective tissue diseases, and heredofamilial diseases.

359. The answer is A (1, 2, 3). *(Braunwald, ed 11. pp 1188–1189, 1202–1203, 1521.)* Because the kidney contains regions of hyperosmolality, low pH, and relative hemostasis and anoxia, it is prone to damage in all sickle cell diseases, including sickle trait. Proteinuria and hematuria are common and may be severe enough to cause the nephrotic syndrome and gross hematuria, respectively. The most consistent feature of sickle cell nephropathy, however, is the inability to concentrate urine. While this defect is reversible in children through multiple transfusions, it is not so in adults in whom maximum urinary concentration does not exceed 400 mOsm/L. Both cortical and medullary necrosis occur and papillary necrosis is not uncommon. There is progressive loss of glomerular filtration rate, but azotemia to the point of requiring dialysis does not occur.

360. The answer is B (1, 3). *(Braunwald, ed 11. p 1180–1181. Ponticelli, Kidney Int 29:927–940, 1986.)* Membranous glomerulonephropathy, a common cause of the nephrotic syndrome, is characterized by diffuse thickening of glomerular capillary walls and subepithelial deposits of immune complexes. Along with the idiopathic variety, frequent causes of this lesion include systemic lupus erythematosus; drugs, most commonly captopril, gold, and penicillamine; neoplasia; and infections, particularly streptococcal, hepatitis B, and syphilis. The most common associated tumor is of the lung. Therapy for membranous glomerulonephropathy is controversial. Recent trials seem to suggest that therapy with steroids and alkylating agents may enhance the natural history of this lesion toward spontaneous resolution. In children, spontaneous complete remissions are common, but they occur in only 20 to 25 percent of adults. In patients undergoing renal transplantation, only rarely has membranous glomerulopathy recurred.

361. The answer is A (1, 2, 3). *(Blandy, pp 362–365. Braunwald, ed 11. p 1203.)* Renal vein thrombosis may be secondary to a variety of causes. In children, dehydration from diarrhea and vomiting associated with gastroenteritis may precipitate renal vein thrombosis. Renal tumors (hypernephromas) may invade the renal veins and result in thrombosis. The thrombotic process, which frequently is heralded by flank pain, hematuria, and proteinuria, may affect both kidneys. Treatment of this disorder may include anticoagulation therapy, thrombectomy, and nephrectomy—if the process is unilateral.

362. The answer is E (all). *(Braunwald, ed 11. pp 1582–1584.)* By whatever method, prostatectomy may lead to a number of complications. Urinary incontinence secondary to external sphincter injury may be devastating. Retrograde ejaculation secondary to resection of the vesical neck is very common and may produce sterility. Urethral stricture formation may result from faulty surgical technique such as inadequate lubrication, prolonged instrumentation, or use of oversized instruments. Epididymitis may also develop; it can be unilateral or bilateral, and its incidence may be lessened by performing a vasectomy prior to prostatectomy.

363. The answer is A (1, 2, 3). *(Braunwald, ed 11. p 1205.)* Polycystic renal disease is generally divided into the adult and infantile forms. The latter is often associated with cysts of the liver and spleen, and death in the neonatal period is not unusual. The adult type commonly becomes manifest after the age of 30; affected patients may present with flank pain and hematuria. Work-up of patients in whom polycystic disease is suspected may reveal markedly enlarged kidneys and hypertension; renal insufficiency commonly ensues. General treatment should be directed to control of the hypertension and management of the renal insufficiency. Death from rupture of cerebral aneurysms occurs in approximately 10 percent of affected patients. Whereas the infantile form is inherited as an autosomal recessive trait, the adult familial form is an autosomal dominant trait.

364. The answer is C (2, 4). *(Blandy, pp 774–781. Braunwald, ed 11. pp 1220–1221.)* Carcinoma of the urinary bladder is generally of the transitional cell variety. It commonly presents with painless hematuria, which may be gross in nature. A high incidence of bladder tumors is reported in those who smoke cigarettes heavily and in people exposed to certain industrial chemical agents such as benzidine, xenyl-amine, and 1- and 2-naphthylamines. Metastatic tumors to the bladder from another primary site are not common.

365–368. The answers are: 365-B, 366-B, 367-B, 368-A. *(Rose, pp 410–411.)* Medullary sponge kidney is characterized by dilation of the terminal collecting ducts to cystic proportions. The cysts are usually diffuse and bilateral, although unilateral changes may be seen; they frequently contain calcium oxalate calculi. Infection and hematuria occur in approximately one-third of patients, while frank renal failure is rare. Hypertension is no more common than in the general population. Many patients with medullary sponge kidney are asymptomatic and the diagnosis is frequently made on intravenous urography performed for some other reason; the disorder is found in 1 of 200 unselected intravenous pyelograms.

Medullary cystic disease is characterized by cystic changes located primarily in the medulla and corticomedullary region, although they may be localized to the collecting ducts and distal convoluted tubules. It is a rare disorder of children that progresses to end-stage renal failure. Familial juvenile nephronophthisis, another condition that develops at somewhat older age, is histologically and clinically similar to medullary cystic disease. While evidence for genetic transmission is lacking in most patients with medullary sponge kidney, the mode of inheritance in medullary cystic kidney disease may be autosomal recessive, autosomal dominant, and X-linked; sporadic forms have been described. The urinalysis is typically normal; however, as tubular function deteriorates, there is a progressive loss of concentrating ability. Polyuria, progressive renal failure, stunted growth, anemia, and hyper-chloremic metabolic acidosis characterize the clinical course of the disease.

369–373. The answers are: 369-B, 370-B, 371-B, 372-C, 373-C. *(Braunwald, ed 11. pp 1439–1440.)* Polyarteritis nodosa (PAN) is a multisystem, necrotizing vasculitis of small- and medium-sized muscular arteries; involvement of the renal and visceral arteries is characteristic. Patients usually present with weakness, ma-laise, headache, myalgias, and abdominal pain as well as with specific complaints relating to involved organs. In over one-half of cases, fever, weight loss, and malaise are present. Anemia, leukocytosis, and hypergammaglobulinemia are commonly seen. Arteriograms may reveal characteristic pathology, such as aneurysms of small- and medium-sized muscular arteries of the kidneys and abdominal viscera. Diagnosis is usually based on the demonstration of vasculitis on biopsy material of involved organs.

Churg-Strauss disease (or syndrome) is a multisystem granulomatous vasculitis of small- and medium-sized muscular arteries, capillaries, veins, and venules; tissue infiltration with eosinophils is commonly present. In contrast to PAN, lung involvement is predominant and there exists a strong association with asthma and peripheral eosinophilia. In addition to fever, malaise, and weight loss, pulmonary findings dominate the clinical picture with the presence of severe asthma and pulmonary infiltrates; otherwise, the multisystem involvement is similar to that seen in PAN but with less common and less severe renal disease.

Oncology and Hematology

DIRECTIONS: Each question below contains five suggested responses. Select the **one best** response to each question.

Polycythemia vera

374. Oncogenes are genes that can mediate oncogenesis. All the following statements about oncogenes are correct EXCEPT that

(A) oncogenes were detected among the chromosomes of 60 percent of normal subjects studied

(B) RNA retroviruses may release oncogenes from normal feedback restraint

(C) patients at risk for oncogene activation and the subsequent development of a T-cell leukemia have been identified in Japan

(D) at least two sets of oncogenes have been described, one that immortalizes the cell while the other completes its transformation

(E) evidence suggests that retroviruses may incorporate a cellular oncogene in one cell and then move to another and insert the cancer-promoting gene into the DNA of the infected cell

375. A 57-year-old white man is found on physical examination to be plethoric with mild splenomegaly and no evidence of chronic cardiac or pulmonary disease. Laboratory examination reveals a hematocrit of 62%, a white cell count of 24,000/mm³, and thrombocytosis. Red blood cell mass was found to be elevated as determined by isotope dilution. True statements concerning this patient's condition include each of the following EXCEPT

(A) 2 percent of patients without prior therapy experience transformation to acute leukemia

(B) there is an increased incidence of peptic ulcer disease

(C) repeated phlebotomies resolve the associated splenomegaly

(D) urine levels of erythropoietin are substantially reduced

(E) pruritus, particularly after bathing, is a frequent complaint

376. Vitamin B_{12} deficiency and therapy are characterized by all the following statements EXCEPT

(A) neurologic symptoms may precede changes in hematocrit
(B) the first stage of the Schilling test is abnormal in patients with intestinal bacterial overgrowth
(C) hypokalemia is a common consequence of vitamin B_{12} therapy
(D) along with megaloblastic changes, the marrow ratio of myeloid precursors to erythroid precursors falls to 1:1
(E) reticulocytosis begins on the third to fifth day of vitamin B_{12} therapy

377. Myelophthisic anemias are characterized by a peripheral blood smear containing all the following EXCEPT

(A) giant platelets
(B) spur cells (acanthocytes)
(C) nucleated red cells
(D) immature granulocytes
(E) teardrop cells (dacryocytes)

378. All the following drugs are contraindicated in patients with glucose-6-phosphate dehydrogenase deficiency EXCEPT

(A) sulfapyridine
(B) nitrofurantoin
(C) colchicine
(D) sulfamethoxazole
(E) phenylhydrazine

379. All the following statements concerning benign monoclonal gammopathy are true EXCEPT

(A) 10 percent of patients will develop multiple myeloma
(B) it is the result of a single clone of B lymphocytes
(C) osteolysis does not occur
(D) the defect in humoral immunity leads to an increased incidence of infection with encapsulated organisms
(E) renal tubular dysfunction may occur secondary to light-chain excretion

380. Aplastic anemia, a condition in which an acellular or markedly hypocellular bone marrow results in pancytopenia, may be caused by all the following EXCEPT

(A) systemic lupus erythematosus
(B) infectious hepatitis
(C) paroxysmal cold hemoglobinuria
(D) paroxysmal nocturnal hemoglobinuria
(E) pregnancy

381. A 12-year-old boy, previously in perfect health, suffers a traumatic rupture of the spleen in an automobile accident. He undergoes an emergency splenectomy. All the following sequelae would be expected EXCEPT

(A) normal splenic function 1 year later
(B) the appearance of intracellular Heinz bodies in the peripheral blood
(C) a white blood cell count of 20,000/mm^3
(D) overwhelming infection with *Haemophilus influenzae*
(E) a temporary requirement for anticoagulant therapy

DIRECTIONS: Each question below contains four suggested responses of which **one or more** is correct. Select

A	if	**1, 2, and 3**	are correct
B	if	**1 and 3**	are correct
C	if	**2 and 4**	are correct
D	if	**4**	is correct
E	if	**1, 2, 3, and 4**	are correct

382. True statements concerning prostate cancer and its treatment include that

(1) bone metastases are uniformly osteoblastic
(2) 95 percent are adenocarcinomas
(3) radiation therapy rarely causes impotence
(4) histologically, tumors are frequently multifocal

383. True statements concerning patients with sickle cell anemia include which of the following?

(1) Newborn infants are protected from the clinical manifestations of the disease during the first several months of life
(2) One-half of adults have bilirubin gallstones
(3) Two-thirds of patients who have one stroke will have at least one more
(4) Dehydration, a precipitating factor of sickle crisis, is likely to occur as patients are unable to concentrate urine above 400 mOsm/L

384. Correct statements concerning drug-induced hemolytic anemia include that

(1) 10 percent of patients taking alpha methyldopa will develop a Coombs-positive hemolytic anemia
(2) quinidine-induced hemolytic anemia is seen only during administration of high doses of the drug
(3) hemolytic anemia secondary to penicillin usually begins during the first 3 days of administration
(4) patients with a history of hemolytic anemia to penicillin have an increased likelihood of developing a hemolytic anemia to cephalosporins

385. In diagnosing iron deficiency anemia, it is correct to say that

(1) absence of detectable iron stored in the marrow occurs early in the development of iron deficiency
(2) mean corpuscular hemoglobin concentration will fall before mean corpuscular volume
(3) measurement of serum ferritin provides a reliable estimate of iron storage and may remove the necessity for bone marrow examination
(4) successful iron replacement can be monitored by the reticulocyte response, which should increase within 3 days of commencing therapy

386. Hemophilia is a genetically transmitted bleeding disorder (sex-linked recessive pattern) characterized by a deficiency in the procoagulant activities of factor VIII. Correct statements about this condition include which of the following?

(1) Males with the disorder transmit the gene to all their daughters, and neither daughters nor sons will have a bleeding tendency

(2) Fifty percent of female carriers can be detected at a 95 percent confidence level

(3) In 30 percent of cases no family history can be elicited

(4) Hemophilia has an incidence of 1 in 100,000 of the population

387. The American Cancer Society guidelines for cancer screening include which of the following recommendations?

(1) Base-line mammography for all women between the ages of 35 and 40

(2) A digital rectal examination every 2 years after age 40

(3) A professional breast examination every year for women over 40

(4) A pelvic examination every 3 years for women over 50

388. A 20-year-old man is being investigated for severe normocytic normochromic anemia (hematocrit 28%). Mild granulocytopenia and thrombocytopenia are present. The patient is found to have hemosiderinuria but no hemoglobinuria. He has a low leukocyte alkaline phosphatase level and a low red blood cell acetylcholinesterase level. Management of this condition should include

(1) corticosteroid treatment

(2) whole blood transfusions

(3) administration of heparin

(4) administration of fluoxymesterone, 20 to 30 mg/day

DIRECTIONS: Each group of questions below consists of lettered headings followed by a set of numbered items. For each numbered item select the **one** lettered heading with which it is **most** closely associated. Each lettered heading may be used **once, more than once, or not at all.**

Questions 389–393

Match the descriptions below with the appropriate pathologic inclusions.

(A) Howell-Jolly bodies
(B) Pappenheimer bodies
(C) Cabot rings (ring bodies)
(D) Heinz bodies
(E) Coarse basophilic stippling

389. Seen in splenectomized patients and in those with hemolytic anemia

390. Seen in reticulocytes in megaloblastic anemia; origin unknown

391. Represent iron granulations

392. Represent an intracellular precipitate of abnormal hemoglobin

393. Represent aggregated ribosomes; characteristic of lead intoxication and thalassemia

Questions 394–398

Match the following.

(A) Methotrexate
(B) Cytosine arabinoside (cytarabine)
(C) Nitrogen mustard
(D) Cyclophosphamide
(E) Doxorubicin

394. A synthetic alkylating agent that must be activated by the mixed function oxidases in hepatic microsomes. Hydration and adequate urinary flow help to prevent cystitis resulting from this drug

395. A synthetic alkylating agent that, being very reactive in aqueous solution, must be used within minutes of solubilization. May cause a severe chemical burn (cellulitis) if, when injected intravenously, it extravasates into subcutaneous tissues

396. A folic acid antagonist that is excreted by the kidneys essentially unchanged. Renal function must be assessed, therefore, prior to use. Chronic use may produce hepatic cirrhosis

397. An antitumor antibiotic that is very useful in the treatment of the lymphomas, sarcomas, acute leukemia, and breast cancer. Chronic use may produce fatal cardiomyopathy

398. An antimetabolite particularly effective against acute leukemia. Dose-limiting effects include nausea, vomiting, and bone marrow depression. Striking megaloblastosis may occur

DIRECTIONS: Each group of questions below consists of four lettered headings followed by a set of numbered items. For each numbered item select

A	if the item is associated with	(A) **only**
B	if the item is associated with	(B) **only**
C	if the item is associated with	**both** (A) and (B)
D	if the item is associated with	**neither** (A) nor (B)

Each lettered heading may be used **once, more than once, or not at all.**

Questions 399–403

(A) Benign gastric ulcer
(B) Malignant gastric ulcer
(C) Both
(D) Neither

399. Affected patients may present with epigastric distress, easy fatigability, anemia, and guaiac-positive stools

400. Affected patients respond to antacid therapy both symptomatically and roentgenographically

401. Affected patients may be genetically predisposed

402. Differential diagnosis includes lymphoma, pseudolymphoma, and Ménétrier's disease

403. Disease may be associated with elevated carcinoembryonic antigen titers

Questions 404–408

(A) Gaucher's disease, adult type
(B) Niemann-Pick disease
(C) Both
(D) Neither

404. Prenatal diagnosis may be established

405. Foam histiocytes characteristic

406. Splenomegaly

407. Skeletal lesions

408. Elevated serum acid phosphatase

Questions 409–413

(A) Chronic myelogenous leukemia (CML)
(B) Agnogenic myeloid metaplasia (AMM)
(C) Both
(D) Neither

409. Increase in the absolute basophil count

410. Absent leukocyte alkaline phosphatase

411. Philadelphia chromosome

412. Osteosclerosis

413. Tendency toward a chronic phase over many years

Questions 414–418

(A) Myasthenia gravis
(B) Myasthenic syndrome (Eaton-Lambert syndrome)
(C) Both
(D) Neither

414. Thymoma

415. Small-cell carcinoma of the lung

416. Physiologic defect at the neuromuscular junction

417. Possible response to neostigmine by affected patients

418. Possible response to guanidine hydrochloride by affected patients

Questions 419–423

    (A) Abnormal prothrombin time (PT)
    (B) Abnormal partial thromboplastin time (PTT)
    (C) Both
    (D) Neither

C 419. Vitamin K deficiency

C 420. Fibrinogen deficiency

B 421. Thrombocytopenia

A 422. Factor VII deficiency

B 423. Factor VIII deficiency

Questions 424–428

    (A) Sideroblastic anemia
    (B) Anemia of chronic disease
    (C) Both
    (D) Neither

C 424. Elevated serum ferritin

B 425. Decreased serum iron

C 426. Increased erythrocyte protoporphyrin

A 427. Erythroid hyperplasia

D 428. Effective iron supplementation

Questions 429–433

    (A) Thrombotic thrombocytopenic purpura (TTP)
    (B) Chronic idiopathic thrombocytopenic purpura (chronic ITP)
    (C) Both
    (D) Neither

C 429. Normal or increased numbers of megakaryocytes

C 430. Steroid therapy

A 431. Fever

A 432. Fragmented red cells

B 433. Elevated levels of platelet-associated IgG in 90 percent of patients

Questions 434–438

    (A) Acute lymphocytic leukemia
    (B) Acute myelocytic leukemia
    (C) Both
    (D) Neither

A 434. Most frequent in children and may be curable

C 435. Usually fatal within 3 months if the affected patient is untreated or fails to respond to therapy, although in individual cases the course of disease can be quite variable

B 436. Histochemical tests are useful in determining morphologic subtypes. Affected cells usually stain positively with peroxidase and Sudan black stain and are negative for para-aminosalicylic acid stain

C 437. Chromosomal abnormalities occur and are diagnostic

B 438. Treatment requires a strategy of intensive chemotherapy that renders affected patients severely hypoplastic or aplastic for a period of time, calling for intensive supportive care

Oncology and Hematology

Answers

374.   The answer is A. *(Braunwald, ed 11. pp 310–315. Rawley, Nature 301:290, 1983.)* The apparently unrelated facts that a number of malignant states are associated with well-defined chromosomal abnormalities (e.g., the Philadelphia chromosome in chronic myeloid leukemia) and that initiating factors could precipitate a malignancy (ionizing radiation, viral infection) can now be brought together with the discovery of oncogenes. This genetic material is found in normal chromosomes so that everyone must be presumed to be at risk for developing cancer should the oncogenes be activated. The best evidence would suggest that oncogenes are normally kept in an inactive state by regulatory genes situated on either side of this cancer-promoting information. Damage to chromosomes, such as that produced by radiation or perhaps an RNA retrovirus, may release the oncogene from these inhibitory influences and activation may follow. At least two sets of oncogenes have been identified and appear to be important. One is involved in promoting the repeated division of cells that leads to their immortality while the other is associated with the completion of the transformation of the cell from its normal to a malignant state. The human T-cell leukemia virus is a retrovirus than can activate oncogenes to produce T-cell leukemia. It is a common form of leukemia in Japan, the West Indies, and now the southeastern part of the United States. In Japan it has been possible to identify those subjects who were at risk for having oncogene activation occur after viral infection. This should allow for prophylactic and early treatment responses to be made that may block the development of this highly malignant tumor. Numerous mechanisms for activation of oncogenes have been proposed, but there is evidence to suggest that one of those mechanisms involves retroviruses incorporating cellular oncogene material and then taking this material to a new cell where malignant proliferation will be induced.

375.   The answer is C. *(Braunwald, ed 11. pp 1529–1531.)* Polycythemia vera is a chronic and progressive disease characterized by an increased production of myeloid elements and splenomegaly. In distinction to the secondary forms of polycythemia, urine and serum levels of erythropoietin are substantially reduced or absent. Because of the increased red blood cell mass, the hemoglobin concentration, hematocrit, and total blood volume are all elevated. Symptoms relating to the associated increased viscosity and reduced cerebral perfusion include headache, head fullness, tinnitus, visual alterations, and syncope. Peripheral vascular symptoms are common and the incidence of peptic ulcer disease is increased. Early satiety and abdominal fullness are related to the associated splenomegaly. Bleeding is common. Laboratory findings include an elevated hemoglobin concentration, leukocytosis with an increase in the absolute basophil count, thrombocytosis, and a very low erythrocyte sedimentation rate. Bone marrow examination reveals either erythroid hyperplasia or panhyperplasia. Progression to marrow fibrosis occurs in 15 to 20 percent of patients and the majority of patients die of vascular complications; acute leukemia will develop in 2 percent of patients. Therapy includes multiple phlebotomies, ^{32}P, and chemotherapy. The initial use of phlebotomy is to reduce the red blood cell mass and blood volume; a hematocrit or hemoglobin value in the low-to-normal range should be the end point of therapy with phlebotomy.

376. The answer is B. *(Williams, ed 3. pp 434–456.)* Vitamin B$_{12}$ deficiency is a cause of megaloblastic anemia and is usually the consequence of abnormal absorption. Because proper utilization of the vitamin depends on its binding with gastric intrinsic factor and an intact distal ileum, any process that interferes with either arm of this scheme will lead to a deficient state. Causes include pernicious anemia, gastrectomy, sprue, fish tapeworm infestations, Crohn's disease, ileal resection, and bacterial overgrowth. Poor dietary intake and states of increased and impaired utilization will also lead to a vitamin B$_{12}$ deficiency state. Helpful in the differential diagnosis of the anemia is the Schilling test. The first stage of the test determines whether a deficiency exists and the second stage determines whether the deficiency is intrinsic-factor dependent. Because an overgrowth of intestinal bacteria competes with the host for both bound and unbound vitamin B$_{12}$, the second stage of the test remains abnormal. Patients may present with glossitis, symptoms of anemia, and neurologic abnormalities, which include numbness and paresthesias in the extremities, ataxia, and disturbance in mentation. The neurologic dysfunction may occur in the presence of a normal hematocrit. With vitamin B$_{12}$ replacement, marrow morphology begins to convert from megaloblastic to erythroblastic and all symptoms are reversed except those attributed to permanent neuronal damage.

377. The answer is B. *(Williams, ed 3. pp 273–274, 528–531.)* Myelophthisic anemia is caused by marrow infiltration due most commonly to lymphoid malignancies and metastatic carcinoma. It is a mild-to-moderate anemia characterized by the premature release of myeloid and erythroid cells from the marrow; indeed, the finding of immature white cells and nucleated red cells in a patient with a known malignancy most probably indicates marrow involvement. The diagnosis of myelophthisic anemia rests on bone biopsy as aspiration of marrow is usually not possible owing to a packed marrow. Myelofibrosis, sclerosis, and significant hypersplenism may accompany the myelophthisic process. Treatment is directed toward the underlying disease, although splenectomy in those with hypersplenism and androgen or steroid therapy for patients with myelofibrosis may cause an improvement in anemia.

378. The answer is C. *(Williams, ed 3. pp 561–569.)* Glucose-6-phosphate dehydrogenase (G6PD) deficiency is a hereditary disease characterized by a decreased
activity of the enzyme and the consequent predisposition of red cells to hemolyze
as a result of drugs, infection, or acidosis. Drug-induced hemolysis results from the
complexing of oxidized glutathione to hemoglobin, which precipitates as Heinz
bodies. Red cells containing these inclusions are rapidly removed from the circulation and hemolysis ensues. There are several types of G6PD deficiency and the
severity of the drug-induced hemolytic anemia is different for each; furthermore,
people with the same G6PD variant will exhibit different degrees of hemolysis to
the same drug. Other than the drugs mentioned in the question—excluding colchicine—the medications to be avoided include pentaquine, primaquine, sulfanilamide,
and nalidixic acid. Treatment of severe hemolysis includes blood transfusions, maintenance of good urine flow, and the administration of vitamin E.

379. The answer is D. *(Williams, ed 3. pp 966–968.)* Benign monoclonal gammopathy is the most common disorder of immunoglobulins and is due to the proliferation of a single B lymphocyte that reaches a steady-state of less than 1×10^{11}
total cells. There is no evidence of neoplasia so that bone destruction, marrow
depression, and a susceptibility to infection are not seen. The syndrome is found
incidentally. Laboratory values are unremarkable although a drop in alternative levels
of immunoglobulin may occur, and marrow plasma cell concentration is normal.
While most patients remain asymptomatic, a minority will go on to develop multiple
myeloma. No therapy is indicated for this syndrome.

380. The answer is C. *(Braunwald, ed 11. pp 1533–1536.)* Failure of stem cell
differentiation in the bone marrow results in pancytopenia, which involves a lack of
erythrocytes, neutrophils, and platelets. The term aplastic anemia should be restricted
to states involving this degree of hypocellularity. A few patients appear to develop
aplastic anemia because of immunologic mechanisms that lead to the destruction of
bone marrow stem cells or prevent their normal maturation. Such mechanisms may
be operative in the infrequent, but well-described, aplastic anemia associated with
active systemic lupus erythematosus. It is of interest that immunoregulatory T cells,
which are disordered in this condition, have also been demonstrated to be capable
of influencing erythroid precursor-cell maturation. Both infectious hepatitis A and
serum hepatitis B may be associated with the development of aplastic anemia, a
complication that is not necessarily related to the severity of the hepatitis and that
usually develops as the hepatitis is resolving. Aplastic anemia is an extremely dangerous complication of hepatitis; in many affected patients the bone marrow suppression is reported to be profound and irreversible. Aplastic anemia can develop in the
course of paroxysmal nocturnal hemoglobinuria and as a complication of pregnancy.
In the latter condition, the bone marrow suppression may remit following delivery
of the fetus. Paroxysmal cold hemoglobinuria today is a rare disorder; formerly, it
occurred in association with tertiary syphilis as a result of the formation of an IgG

antibody directed against the P antigen on the surface of red blood cells. Now that syphilis has again become prevalent, paroxysmal cold hemoglobinuria also may reappear with increasing frequency. Rarely, idiopathic cases of paroxysmal cold hemoglobinuria may occur, but such cases have not been associated with the development of an aplastic anemia.

381. The answer is D. *(Braunwald, ed 11. p 277.)* Removal of a spleen that has been damaged by traumatic rupture is a common surgical procedure; thus, significant data exist concerning the effects of this operation on host defense mechanisms. Of the numerous sequelae that follow, an increase in susceptibility to infection following removal of the spleen in patients with diseases of that organ is not a common one. Thus, it would be surprising to have an otherwise healthy child overcome by *Haemophilus influenzae* infection. The hematological changes associated with removal of all splenic function, mainly the appearance of red blood cells with Howell-Jolly bodies, acanthocytes and siderocytes, Heinz bodies, and target cells all would be expected. Normal splenic function may be found in patients within a year of splenectomy. In many instances this restoration of function will be due to the presence of an accessory spleen that has appropriately hypertrophied; recent evidence, however, would suggest that, in the vast majority of children who undergo splenectomy, rudimentary splenic tissue present in all people expands into a functioning organ. Within 2 weeks of surgery, a leukocytosis of 20,000/mm^3 and a thrombocytosis exceeding 1,000,000/mm^3 are not uncommon. Because a steep rise in platelet count can be associated with portal vein thrombosis, prophylactic anticoagulant therapy should be instituted if the platelet level approaches this figure.

382. The answer is C (2, 4). *(Braunwald, ed 11. pp 1582–1585.)* Prostate cancers, which are most commonly adenocarcinomas, are the second most common malignancy in men. They may spread by direct extension, hematogenously, or via the lymphatics, and commonly cause both osteoblastic and osteoclastic bone metastases. Staging is divided into four main groups with stages A and B designating tumor confined to the prostate and stages C and D tumor spread beyond the capsule. Treatment for cancer of the prostate involves surgery, radiation therapy, androgen therapy, and chemotherapy in various combinations dependent on the type and stage of the tumor. In patients receiving external beam radiation, 30 to 60 percent suffer impotence.

383. The answer is E (all). *(Williams, ed 3. pp 589–596.)* A patient with sickle cell anemia is homozygous for the gene for sickle hemoglobin and will, after the first few months of life and as the level of fetal hemoglobin falls, suffer the consequences of sickling red blood cells. Bone pain, aseptic necrosis of the head of the femur, renal papillary necrosis, priapism, skin ulcers, gallstones, pulmonary infarctions, retinal detachment, and cerebrovascular accidents can all result from sickling and hemolyzing red cells. Because of repeated infarctions, there is marked impairment of splenic function both in terms of antibody production and phagocytic activity, thereby allowing for an increased susceptibility to infection with encapsulated organisms. Laboratory studies reveal a microcytic anemia with a reticulocytosis, increased levels of indirect bilirubin, and, usually, a leukocytosis and thrombocytosis even in the asymptomatic patient. Diagnosis is made by hemoglobin electrophoresis. Therapy involves hydration, transfusions of red blood cells, folic acid supplementation, and prophylaxis with pneumococcal vaccine.

384. The answer is D (4). *(Williams, ed 3. pp 648–650.)* Three mechanisms explain the pathogenesis of drug-induced hemolytic anemia. In the immune complex mechanism characterized by quinidine, isoniazid, sulfonamides, and phenacetin, the drug combines with preformed antibody. The resultant complexes bind reversibly to red cells, which are then hemolyzed by fixed complement. Only small amounts of drug are needed for hemolysis because the immune complexes are capable of migrating from cell to cell. Alpha methyldopa, in contrast, seems to cause a hemolytic anemia by inactivating suppressor-cell function, allowing autoantibodies to form against red-cell antigens. Fully 10 percent of people taking alpha methyldopa will be Coombs-positive but less than 1 percent will experience a hemolytic anemia, usually 3 to 6 months after initiating therapy. In hapten-mediated anemia, the involved drug coats circulating red cells and is then bound by specific antibody; the immune complex-coated erythrocytes are destroyed through splenic sequestration. Penicillin and the cephalosporins (which have antigenic cross-reactivity with penicillin) are prime examples of this type of hemolytic anemia, which begins after 7 to 10 days of drug use.

385. The answer is B (1, 3). *(Braunwald, ed 11. pp 1495–1497.)* Patients with chronic conditions such as rheumatoid arthritis often have a low serum iron level, whereas their total iron stores, as seen in a marrow biopsy, are within normal limits. In genuinely iron-deficient patients, no stainable iron will be present in marrow tissue. As total iron body stores fall, corpuscular volume decreases and, in a more chronic stage, mean corpuscular hemoglobin concentration falls. The need for pursuing bone marrow tissue has been reduced by the finding that serum ferritin levels correlate extremely well with tissue stores of iron. In severe cases of iron deficiency anemia, serum ferritin levels may fall by as much as 90 percent. In such cases, free erythrocyte porphyrin is usually elevated. The mainstay of therapy for iron deficiency anemia continues to be ferrous sulfate. It is important to follow the progress of the therapy during the first 10 days with serial reticulocyte counts. Reticulocytosis can be expected after the seventh, and before the tenth, day of replacement therapy with ferrous sulfate.

386. The answer is A (1, 2, 3). *(Braunwald, ed 11. pp 1476–1477.)* With the improved treatment for hemophilia, it is theoretically possible that a growing number of affected males could pass the abnormal gene on to their progeny. Inasmuch as sex (or the lack of femaleness) is determined by the male Y chromosome, all sons of men with hemophilia will be normal. However, all daughters of such patients will possess the abnormal genes. Thus, the major emphasis continues to be placed on the detection of female carriers. Hemophilia follows the sex-linked inheritance pattern. Mothers may expect 50 percent of their sons to be affected by the disease and 50 percent of their daughters to carry the abnormal gene. Fortunately, it is now possible with a high degree of accuracy to detect female carriers. The test involves the determination of both the antigenicity of factor VIII in suspected carriers as well as the serum level of functional factor VIII. By examining both properties of factor VIII, 30 percent of carriers can be detected at the 99 percent level of confidence and at least 50 percent at the 95 percent confidence level. Spontaneous mutations on the X chromosome obviously occur, for as many as 30 percent of hemophiliacs have no family history of the disease. Of the inherited disturbances in coagulation, hemophilia is the most common—it affects 1 in every 10,000 births.

387.   The answer is B (1, 3).   *(Braunwald, ed 11. p 430. CA 30:194, 1980.)* The study of risk factors for the development of various forms of cancer is the basis for the guidelines for early detection developed by the American Cancer Society. The guidelines have remained unchanged since 1980 and are age-related:

20 to 40 years of age
—a cancer-related check-up every 3 years
—a professional breast examination every 3 years; a self examination every month; and a base-line mammography between the ages of 35 and 40
—a pelvic examination every 3 years
—a Pap test every 3 years after two negative yearly examinations
40 years of age and over
—a yearly cancer check-up
—a professional breast examination every year; a self-examination every month; and mammography every 1 to 2 years for women 40 to 49 years of age and every year for those 50 and over
—a pelvic examination every year
—a Pap test every 3 years after two negative yearly examinations
—an endometrial tissue sample at menopause in a patient with high risk factors
—a yearly digital rectal examination after age 40; a yearly stool occult blood test after 50; and a sigmoidoscopic examination every 3 years after two negative yearly examinations after age 50

Chest x-rays and sputum cytology are no longer recommended even for people at high risk for the development of lung cancer.

388. The answer is C (2, 4). *(Braunwald, ed 11. pp 1513–1514.)* The patient presented in the question suffers from paroxysmal nocturnal hemoglobinuria (PNH). Notwithstanding the name of the syndrome, hemoglobinuria is seldom gross and may occur only intermittently—in some affected patients no more than trace amounts may ever occur. Similarly, the anemia associated with this condition is variable, being profound in only a few patients. Most patients exhibit normal levels of hemoglobin or only moderate reductions. The diagnosis, however, would be extremely unlikely in the absence of hemosiderin in the urine. A preliminary diagnosis of PNH is confirmed with an acid hemolysis test or sucrose lysis test. Further confirmation would be evidence of low concentrations of leukocyte alkaline phosphatase and red blood cell acetylcholinesterase. Activation of the terminal part of the complement cascade normally is associated with some red blood cell lysis. However, patients with PNH are inordinately sensitive to these complement components. In addition to erythrocytes, granulocytes and platelets also are sensitive to these mechanisms. Transfusions of whole blood are usually beneficial. Although blood transfusions will contain some complement components and their substrates, this potential danger is offset by the passive increase in hemoglobin levels that follows transfusion. The increase in hemoglobin will suppress bone marrow production of young erythrocytes, which are particularly sensitive to complement. For similar reasons, the administration of ferrous sulfate to promote increased erythropoiesis will lead to the production of excessive numbers of young erythrocytes that will be destroyed by complement. Therapy with androgens, such as fluoxymesterone, frequently decreases the destruction of red blood cells and allows hemoglobin levels to rise. These steroids have been shown to affect both complement and red blood cells; however, their mechanism of action in this disease is not certain. PNH frequently is complicated by venous thromboses, for which prophylactic anticoagulation will be necessary. Coumarin-type drugs are useful in such situations, but heparin, which has been found actually to increase the rate of hemolysis, should be avoided.

389–393. The answers are: 389-A, 390-C, 391-B, 392-D, 393-E. *(Williams, ed 3. pp 270–271.)* Pathologic inclusions found in reticulocytes are nuclear or cytoplasmic remnants that are present in various disease states. Howell-Jolly bodies are nuclear remnants that are either chromosomes that have separated from the mitotic spindle during mitosis (the result of nuclear fragmentation) or the product of incomplete nuclear expulsion. They are normally removed during passage through the spleen. Howell-Jolly bodies are found in patients with hemolytic anemia or megaloblastic anemia, and in those who have been splenectomized.

Cabot rings (ring bodies), which usually appear as singular rings in reticulocytes on Wright's-stained film, are found in megaloblastic anemias; their origin is unknown.

Pappenheimer bodies are peripherally located siderosomes and appear as small, dense blue granules on Wright's stain.

Heinz bodies are found in patients with hemoglobin variants. Because of their decreased solubility, these abnormal hemoglobins readily precipitate. Red cells with Heinz bodies are usually pitted or destroyed by the reticuloendothelial system.

Basophilic stippling is also seen in conditions of abnormal hemoglobin biosynthesis and represents aggregates of ribosomes. It is a characteristic feature of lead intoxication and thalassemias.

394–398. The answers are: 394-D, 395-C, 396-A, 397-E, 398-B. *(Braunwald, ed 11. pp 433–437.)* Cyclophosphamide in its commercial form is inactive. It was designed in the hope that its chemical activation would be confined to tumor cells. While this is not the case, cyclophosphamide continues to be a very effective antitumor agent. Although the active antitumor metabolites are unidentified, it is certain that they are excreted in the urine. These metabolites are strongly irritating to the bladder mucosa; their effects range from mild dysuria to severe hemorrhagic cystitis and death. Therefore, normal bladder evacuation and a dilute urine are imperative with the use of cyclophosphamide.

Nitrogen mustard was the first chemotherapeutic agent found to be effective against human cancer. Its major use is in the treatment of lymphoproliferative disorders. Toxic manifestations other than those listed in the question include nausea, vomiting, bone marrow suppression, and alopecia.

Methotrexate was synthesized with the deliberate intent to form a potent folate antagonist because of the observation that exogenous folic acid appeared to accelerate the progression of acute leukemia. The drug has a wide tumoricidal spectrum including acute leukemia, breast cancer, head and neck cancer, choriocarcinoma, and osteogenic sarcoma. Major dose-limiting effects of methotrexate include bone marrow suppression and oral and gastrointestinal toxicity.

Doxorubicin is isolated from *Streptomyces peucetius*. It functions as an inhibitor of DNA synthesis via intercalation into the DNA molecule. Side effects other than cardiotoxicity include nausea, vomiting, bone marrow suppression, alopecia, and stomatitis.

Cytosine arabinoside (also called cytarabine and AraC) is an analogue of the naturally occurring cytosine ribonucleoside. It must be activated via cytidine kinase to the active nucleotide AraCTP, which competes with CTP for the polymerase enzyme. It is particularly effective against acute leukemia. Dose-limiting toxicity includes nausea, vomiting, and bone marrow suppression. Because of its short physical half-life, this agent must be given in multiple repeated injections or as a constant infusion. Oral AraC is ineffective because of the high concentration of cytidine deaminase in the intestinal mucosa that converts AraC to the inactive uracil arabinoside.

399–403. The answers are: 399-C, 400-C, 401-B, 402-B, 403-B. *(Braunwald, ed 11. pp 1246–1247.)* The clinical histories associated with benign and malignant gastric ulcers tend to be quite similar. The peak incidence for benign ulcer disease is between 45 and 55 years of age; for gastric carcinoma, it is 55 years of age. Both benign and malignant ulcer diseases affect men more frequently than women, the ratio being 3.5:1 for the benign disease, and 2:1 for the malignant. While benign gastric ulcer disease does not appear to have a familial predisposition, gastric cancer is two to four times more common in relatives of affected patients than in the general population.

Symptoms of benign gastric ulcers may be quite vague; easy satiety and nausea after eating are common complaints. Midepigastric pain may be aggravated by eating, and weight loss is frequent. Bleeding results in guaiac-positive stools, and secondary anemia and weight loss result in easy fatigability.

Although the clinical history associated with benign gastric ulcers is shared by the majority of patients afflicted with malignant gastric ulcers, approximately 25 percent of such patients present classic *duodenal* ulcer symptoms, including midepigastric burning pain relieved by food.

Preoperative differentiation between benign and malignant ulcer disease is possible in 80 to 90 percent of cases. Radiology can accurately differentiate between them approximately 85 percent of the time. Gastroscopy, cytologic examination, and biopsy of the lesions yield a diagnostic accuracy as high as 90 percent. False positive cytologic results are exceedingly uncommon; most diagnostic errors arise from false negatives. Examination of gastric acid is very helpful; true achlorhydria following maximal pentagastric stimulation almost always excludes a benign gastric ulcer. Yet the presence of acid does not rule out gastric carcinoma. Moreover, improvement in response to medical therapy, both subjectively and on x-ray, can occur in patients who have malignant ulcers. If, following testing, doubt persists as to whether or not the lesion is benign, the affected patient should have surgery.

Conditions that often mimic malignant ulcers on x-ray include peptic ulcer disease, hypertrophic pyloric stenosis, antral gastritis, inflammatory polyps, Ménétrier's disease, lymphoma, pseudolymphoma, Crohn's disease, gastric varices, hematoma, and bezoars or retained food. Unfortunately, carcinoembryonic antigen titers reach diagnostic levels only after cancer has metastasized and, thus, are valueless in early diagnosis.

404–408. The answers are: 404-C, 405-B, 406-C, 407-C, 408-A. *(Williams, ed 3. pp 865–869.)* The lipid storage diseases are hereditary disorders in which lipid accumulates in various tissues. Gaucher's disease, inherited as an autosomal recessive disorder, is caused by a deficiency of β-glucosidase activity with the consequent accumulation of glucocerebroside in spleen, liver, and marrow. Splenomegaly results in mild hemolysis, moderate leukopenia, and severe thrombocytopenia. Liver fibrosis may develop. Bone pain is diffuse as skeletal lesions are widespread. Laboratory features include a normochromic, normocytic anemia, thrombocytopenia, an elevated acid phosphatase, deficient leukocyte β-glucosidase, and various indices of hepatic dysfunction; factor IX deficiency is common and does not relate to the extent of liver disease.

Niemann-Pick disease is inherited as an autosomal recessive disorder and is an affliction of infancy. The disease is due to a deficiency of sphingomyelinase that leads to the accumulation of sphingomyelin throughout the body. The most characteristic histopathologic feature of the disorder is the presence of foam histiocytes. During the first months of life, development is delayed, the abdomen enlarges, and blindness and deafness may ensue. The development of hyporeflexic, flaccid extremities occurs in the second year of life. Bony lesions may be present. There is no effective treatment for Neimann-Pick disease.

409–413. The answers are: 409-C, 410-A, 411-A, 412-B, 413-B. *(Braunwald, ed 11. pp 1527–1529, 1531–1532.)* Both CML and AMM represent neoplasms of the multipotent hematopoietic stem cell. CML is characterized by splenomegaly and increased numbers of granulocytes, particularly neutrophils; the white blood cell count often exceeds 200,000/mm^3. Presenting symptoms are related to splenomegaly, anemia, or hypermetabolism; arthralgias, thrombohemorrhagic complications, and, rarely, lymphadenopathy are also seen. The disorder generally runs a mild course until it transforms into a leukemic phase when the marrow produces increased numbers of blasts and promyelocytes. Laboratory findings include a marked leukocytosis, basophilia, elevated serum B$_{12}$ levels, markedly reduced leukocyte alkaline phosphatase levels, and hyperuricemia. More than 95 percent of patients have the Philadelphia chromosome, which represents a reciprocal translocation of genetic material between the long arms of chromosome 22 and chromosome 9.

AMM is characterized by splenomegaly, progressive fibrosis of bone marrow, and anemia. Fatigue, weakness, anorexia, and symptoms relating to splenomegaly are common presentations. Laboratory abnormalities include an elevated white blood cell count to as high as 50,000/mm^3, an increase in the absolute basophil count, a leukocyte alkaline phosphatase that may be high, normal, or low, and thrombocytopenia. There are no unique cytogenetic abnormalities. Both fibrosis, which is seen in 10 to 15 percent of patients with CML, and osteosclerosis may be found. The disorder generally runs a prolonged course; 25 percent of patients may live 15 years. Transformation to acute leukemia occurs in 5 to 10 percent of patients and may be related to prior therapy.

414–418. The answers are: 414-A, 415-B, 416-C, 417-A, 418-B. *(Braunwald, ed 11. pp 2079–2082.)* Both myasthenia gravis and the myasthenic syndrome (Eaton-Lambert syndrome) may be associated with tumors—the former with lymphoblastic and epithelial tumors of the thymus, the latter with small-cell carcinoma of the lung. Since the myasthenic syndrome may precede the appearance of the tumor by as much as 2 years, and because response to therapy may be quite different for the two myasthenic disorders, they must be carefully distinguished.

Both conditions involve abnormalities at the myoneural junction. However, the conditions can be differentiated on an anatomic, physiologic, and pharmacologic basis, as well as by their association with other morbid conditions. Although myasthenia gravis generally occurs independently of other disorders, 8 to 10 percent of myasthenic patients have a tumor of the thymus gland. Removal of this tumor may result in improvement of the myasthenia gravis. The muscle groups characteristically affected in myasthenia gravis are the facial, oculomotor, laryngeal, pharyngeal, and respiratory. Late in the disease, the shoulder and pelvic muscles also become involved. In contrast, the myasthenic syndrome, which usually spares the bulbar musculature, initially weakens the muscles of the pelvic and shoulder girdles. Each disorder has characteristic electromyographic findings. Myasthenia gravis exhibits a characteristic "myasthenic fatigability" pattern evoked by rapid repetitive stimuli. In the myasthenic syndrome, however, electromyography reveals a recruitment phenomenon involving an initially low amplitude pattern that, with rapid repetitive stimuli, increases.

The edrophonium chloride (Tensilon) test is also helpful in distinguishing myasthenia gravis from the myasthenic syndrome. Tensilon is the preferred cholinesterase antagonist for diagnostic purposes because the response to it is nearly instantaneous and its effect vanishes in minutes. In true myasthenia gravis, Tensilon causes dramatic improvement in muscle strength. Affected patients who so respond to Tensilon can be treated safely with longer-acting cholinesterase inhibitors, such as neostigmine. While cholinesterase inhibitors have little or no effect on the muscle weakness of the myasthenic syndrome, muscle function in this disorder can be dramatically restored either by removing the associated tumor or controlling it with irradiation or chemotherapy, or both. If neither is possible, palliative therapy with guanidine hydrochloride may improve muscle strength. Both groups of affected patients are inordinately sensitive to small doses of tubocurarine and decamethonium.

419–423. The answers are: 419-C, 420-C, 421-D, 422-A, 423-B. *(Williams, ed 3. pp 1263, 1662–1666.)* The prothrombin time and partial thromboplastin time are measures of coagulant activity, the two differing in the branch of the coagulation system tested. The one-stage prothrombin time measures the activity of the extrinsic system, that is, the overall functioning of fibrinogen, prothrombin, and factors V, VII, and X. It is prolonged in any clinical condition (e.g., vitamin K deficiency) that results in a deficiency in any of these factors; prolongation also occurs in the presence of fibrin or fibrinogen-split products and in heparin administration. The PTT is a measure of the functioning of all coagulation factors except VII and XIII. Along with conditions of factor deficiency, it is also abnormal in instances where inhibitors to any of these factors are present; heparin and fibrin or fibrinogen-split products prolong PTT. Any condition that leads to a deficiency in factors measured by both tests will obviously lead to a prolongation of both the PT and PTT.

424–428. The answers are: 424-C, 425-B, 426-C, 427-A, 428-D. *(Braunwald, ed 11. pp 1497–1498, 1504–1506. Williams, ed 3. pp 522–526, 537–544.)* Whether hereditary or acquired, responsive or unresponsive to pyridoxine, the sideroblastic anemias are characterized by hypochromic, microcytic red cells, ineffective erythropoiesis, increased levels of tissue iron, and many ringed sideroblasts in the marrow. In primary sideroblastic anemia, there exists a mitochondrial iron overload secondary to a deficit in the insertion of iron in the porphyrin ring due either to a deficiency of protoporphyrin or globin, or a dysfunction of heme synthetase. Patients usually present in the sixth decade with weakness, fatigue, pallor, and hepatomegaly. The anemia is generally refractory to therapy but, since a small minority of patients do respond, a trial of pyridoxine and folic acid for at least 3 months is worthwhile. The secondary sideroblastic anemias are associated with such conditions as myeloma, hemolytic anemia, Hodgkin's disease, leukemia, rheumatoid arthritis, hypothyroidism, and lead intoxication, and with drugs that interfere with aminolevulinic acid synthetase activity such as isoniazid and chloramphenicol. Alcohol is believed to cause a sideroblastic anemia by inhibiting pyridoxal kinase. Treatment involves removal of the causative condition; when this cannot be done, a trial of pyridoxine and folic acid should be attempted. There are inherited and pyridoxine-responsive forms of sideroblastic anemia, as well.

The anemia of chronic diseases, on the other hand, is characterized by an abnormal iron metabolism, a decreased red cell life span, and an inadequate compensatory marrow response in the setting of a chronic illness. It is also a hypochromic, microcytic anemia and is associated with only a moderate decrease in hemoglobin, a decreased serum iron and total iron binding capacity, and an increased serum ferritin. Proper therapy consists only of transfusions in the symptomatic patient.

429–433. The answers are: 429-C, 430-C, 431-A, 432-A, 433-B. *(Williams, ed 3. pp 1304–1308.)* TTP is characterized by microangiopathic hemolytic anemia, thrombocytopenia, and neurologic dysfunction with the variable presence of fever and renal disease. The disorder may be either chronic or, more commonly, acute. Patients present with fluctuating neurologic abnormalities such as seizures, mental status changes, behavioral disorders, jaundice, purpura, and various manifestations of diffuse microinfarction, such as abdominal pain and complete heart block, caused by widespread hyaline occlusions of small vessels. The peripheral smear is consistent with a microangiopathic hemolytic anemia; thrombocytopenia, hyperbilirubinemia, leukocytosis, proteinuria, and hematuria are other frequent findings. Therapy involves a combination of glucocorticoids, platelet inhibitors, and plasmapheresis and results in remission in 60 to 80 percent of cases.

Chronic ITP, in contrast, is characterized by thrombocytopenia due to immunologically mediated mechanisms. The disease begins insidiously; patients present with petechiae, easy bleeding, hemorrhagic bullae of the oral mucosa, and ecchymosis. Thrombocytopenia, anemia in proportion to blood loss unless a Coombs-positive hemolytic anemia is present, and platelet-associated IgG are typical findings. Only 10 to 20 percent of patients recover spontaneously. Treatment involves the use of steroids to suppress the phagocytic activity of the reticuloendothelial system against the antibody-coated platelets and to decrease antibody synthesis. For those who fail to respond to steroids, splenectomy is performed and improves 70 to 90 percent of patients. Cytotoxic drugs are used in those patients who fail to respond to splenectomy or who are poor surgical risks.

434–438. The answers are: 434-A, 435-C, 436-B, 437-C, 438-B. *(Braunwald, ed 11. pp 1542–1549.)* The peak incidence of acute lymphocytic leukemia (ALL) is between the ages of 2 and 4 years. Although the disease also occurs in adults, adult leukemia is predominantly myelogenous (myelocytic, myelomonocytic, monocytic, promyelocytic, and erythroleukemic). The sexes are equally affected in very young children; however, in older patients, ALL shows a slight male predominance (3:2).

All acute leukemia patients who fail to respond to therapy have a median survival of approximately 3 months. Death usually results from one of the complications of bone marrow failure, i.e., infection or bleeding or both. However, modern therapy allows 90 to 95 percent of children who have ALL to enter remission; the median survival is approximately 5 years. It is projected that 25 percent of these patients may be cured. Acute leukemia therapy is divided into several stages: induction, consolidation, central nervous system prophylaxis, and maintenance. Although approximately 50 percent of patients who have acute myelocytic leukemia (AML) will enter complete remission, the median duration of their remissions is only 10 to 12 months owing to a lack of effective measures to maintain the remission.

It is important to distinguish the two major forms of acute leukemia because the choice of therapy and prognosis in each is quite different. This differentiation can frequently be accomplished by the examination of Wright's-stained smears of the bone marrow. In ALL, the lymphoblasts have a high nuclear:cytoplasmic ratio, scant nucleoli (one or two), and no Auer rods, and the myeloid elements that are present appear normal. The lymphoblasts stain positively with para-aminosalicylic acid (PAS) and negatively with peroxidase and Sudan black. In contrast, leukemic myeloblasts contain more nucleoli (two to four) in a homogeneous "ground glass" nucleus. Auer rods may be evident in the cytoplasm and other more mature myeloid elements may be abnormal. The myeloblasts stain positively with peroxidase and Sudan black and negatively with PAS.

Chromosomal abnormalities may be quite common in the blasts of acute leukemia. Fifty percent of patients who have AML exhibit some chromosomal abnormality in number or structure or both, using standard techniques; these abnormalities vary from patient to patient. With improved techniques, however, according to a recent report, such abnormalities may be far more common than was formerly believed. The only leukemia with a fairly consistent chromosomal abnormality is chronic myelocytic leukemia, in which 90 percent of affected patients have the Philadelphia chromosome.

The four most active drugs for inducing remission in AML are cytosine arabinoside, 6-thioguanine, daunorubicin, and doxorubicin, usually given in combination. Each of these drugs destroys normal stem cells of the bone marrow. Consequently, the anemia, granulocytopenia, and thrombocytopenia that testify to the myelophthisic effects of the disease are severely aggravated by the indiscriminate effects of these drugs. Therefore, during chemotherapy, patients who have AML must receive meticulous supportive care with blood products and antibiotics if the consequences of bone marrow failure are to be ameliorated. In contrast, prednisone, vincristine, and asparaginase, the drugs most capable of inducing remission in children who have ALL, do not destroy the normal myeloid elements of bone marrow.

Neurology

DIRECTIONS: Each question below contains five suggested responses. Select the **one best** response to each question.

439. An 18-year-old man complains to his physician that of late he has developed severe muscle weakness that comes on shortly after he finishes jogging. The attacks are frightening. Only speech and breathing are normal; all other functions requiring a muscular response are extremely weak. His mother adds that the patient's father had a similar problem before being killed in a car accident. All the following would represent an appropriate response on the part of the physician EXCEPT

(A) inquiring about the patient's intake of licorice
(B) obtaining thyroid function tests
(C) checking the patient's potassium level after exercise
(D) checking serum electrolytes between attacks
(E) arranging for a Tensilon test during the next attack

440. A 55-year-old diabetic woman suddenly develops weakness of the left side of her face as well as of her right arm and leg. She also has diplopia on left lateral gaze. The lesion affecting this patient is probably located in the

(A) right cerebral hemisphere
(B) left cerebral hemisphere
(C) right side of the brainstem
(D) left side of the brainstem
(E) right medial longitudinal fasciculus

441. All the following conditions are associated with a delay in reflex relaxation of the Achilles' tendon EXCEPT

(A) pernicious anemia
(B) hypothermia
(C) Addison's disease
(D) quinidine administration
(E) diabetes mellitus

442. All the following statements concerning brain abscess are true EXCEPT

(A) 35 percent of patients require long-term anticonvulsant medication
(B) lumbar puncture is contraindicated in patients with a suspected brain abscess
(C) 40 percent of patients have a normal peripheral white count
(D) fever is present in the vast majority of patients
(E) it is characterized by a ring-enhancing lesion on CT scan

443. A 19-year-old man tells his physician that he has been troubled for 4 days by a severe pain across the top of his right shoulder and the upper part of his right arm. He thought he might have injured the arm but became alarmed when the pain subsided and a progressive weakness developed. All the following comments provoked by this story would be reasonable EXCEPT

(A) he may well have received a tetanus toxoid shot in the arm a week before the trouble started
(B) nerve conduction velocity studies may identify a local brachial plexus disturbance
(C) sensory loss may be as severe as, if not more severe than, the muscle weakness
(D) the patient is likely to have recently had a flulike illness
(E) it would not be surprising if the patient had received an injection of antitoxin within several days before the pain started

444. All the following statements about the treatment of Parkinson's disease are correct EXCEPT

(A) levodopa is usually administered in conjunction with carbidopa
(B) amantadine tends to be beneficial for the tremor associated with the disease
(C) treatment, while ameliorating symptoms, does not alter the natural history of the disease
(D) dyskinesia appears in 20 percent of patients who have received levodopa for more than 1 year
(E) bromocriptine is a useful dopamine receptor agonist

445. A patient arrives at a hospital breathing, but without other evidence of brain function. Two electroencephalograms at 24-hour intervals are isoelectric. A reasonably good chance of full recovery exists if the underlying factor is

(A) cardiac arrest
(B) intracerebral hemorrhage
(C) encephalitis
(D) head trauma
(E) barbiturate overdose

446. Which of the following symptoms would suggest that the headaches suffered by a patient were truly migraine?

(A) A visual field defect that persists as the headache eases
(B) A facial sensory loss in the first division of the trigeminal nerve that coincides with the onset of a severe unilateral headache
(C) A severe headache that is precipitated by a coughing spasm
(D) A first migrainelike attack at the age of 46 years
(E) Migrainelike headaches developing at the same time that birth control pills are started

447. The combination of extensor plantar reflexes and absent ankle reflexes may be due to all the following conditions EXCEPT

(A) vitamin B_{12} deficiency
(B) multiple disc lesions
(C) motor system disease
(D) syringomyelia
(E) tumor of the cauda equina

448. A 45-year-old man, who is a heavy drinker, is admitted to a hospital with diplopia, mild drowsiness, disorientation, and ataxia of a week's duration. On examination, this patient is found to be inattentive and unable to concentrate. He is disoriented in time and place and periodically falls asleep during conversation. He exhibits horizontal and vertical nystagmus and bilateral gaze palsies. Examination of the periphery reveals a symmetrical polyneuropathy. This diagnostic picture is most consistent with which of the following?

(A) Korsakoff's psychosis
(B) Marchiafava-Bignami disease
(C) Wernicke's disease
(D) Wernicke-Korsakoff syndrome
(E) Alcoholic hypoglycemia

449. A 35-year-old man with a history of depression ingests a chemical in an unsuccessful suicide attempt. Twenty-four hours later he becomes blind and his optic discs are noted to be hyperemic. The most probable toxin involved is

(A) isopropyl alcohol
(B) methyl alcohol
(C) carbon tetrachloride
(D) phenol
(E) kerosene

DIRECTIONS: Each question below contains four suggested responses of which **one or more** is correct. Select

A	if	**1, 2, and 3**	are correct
B	if	**1 and 3**	are correct
C	if	**2 and 4**	are correct
D	if	**4**	is correct
E	if	**1, 2, 3, and 4**	are correct

450. A patient suffering from narcolepsy is likely to

(1) have increased periods of REM (rapid eye movement) sleep

(2) experience terrifying hallucinations while awakening

(3) respond to treatment with methylphenidate

(4) have attacks stimulated by emotional or exciting experiences

451. In adult patients with proximal muscle weakness of several months' duration, the differential diagnosis includes polymyositis and the muscular dystrophies. Which of the following would favor the diagnosis of polymyositis?

(1) Markedly elevated creatine kinase (CK) and aldolase levels

(2) Many fibrillation potentials on EMG

(3) Association with other connective tissue diseases

(4) Marked improvement with steroid therapy

452. True statements concerning transient ischemic attacks (TIAs) include which of the following?

(1) TIAs are a predictor of cerebral and myocardial infarctions

(2) Twenty percent of infarcts that follow TIAs occur within 1 month of the first attack

(3) Diplopia, bifacial numbness, and dysarthria imply vertebral-basilar pathology

(4) TIAs of the carotid system commonly involve the eye and brain simultaneously

453. Correct statements concerning trauma-induced seizures include which of the following?

(1) Petit mal seizures occur commonly after trauma

(2) Most are controlled by anticonvulsant medication

(3) The greater the interval between injury and the first seizure, the more likely a complete remission will occur

(4) In the absence of a cerebral contusion or laceration, trauma does not increase the risk of developing seizures

SUMMARY OF DIRECTIONS

A	B	C	D	E
1,2,3	1,3	2,4	4	All are
only	only	only	only	correct

454. True statements concerning pseudotumor cerebri include that

(1) visual field testing commonly shows peripheral constriction
(2) subarachnoid hemorrhage is the most feared complication
(3) it is most commonly found in young, obese women
(4) headaches correlate with elevations in cerebrospinal fluid pressure

455. Correct statements concerning Huntington's chorea include which of the following?

(1) It is associated with a high suicide rate
(2) Wasting of the head of the caudate nucleus and putamen is seen
(3) Patients worsen with the administration of L-dopa
(4) choreoathetosis invariably precedes the manifestations of the psychic disorder

456. The syndrome of inappropriate antidiuretic hormone secretion (SIADH) is associated with which of the following disorders?

(1) Subarachnoid hemorrhage
(2) Meningitis
(3) Guillain-Barré syndrome
(4) Acute encephalitis

457. True statements concerning hypertensive encephalopathy include which of the following?

(1) CSF protein levels are elevated
(2) Symptoms typically include headache, nausea and vomiting, and convulsions
(3) With treatment, symptoms are reversed within 12 to 72 hours
(4) It occurs most often in patients with secondary hypertension

458. Precipitating factors in hepatic encephalopathy include

(1) increased dietary protein
(2) gastrointestinal bleeding
(3) infection
(4) hypokalemic alkalosis

459. Correct statements concerning the pharmacologic evaluation of pupillary innervation include which of the following?

(1) The instillation of a 1:1000 solution of epinephrine into the conjunctival sac will cause the sympathetically denervated pupil to dilate
(2) A normal response to the topical administration of cocaine is pupillary constriction
(3) The denervated pupil will constrict upon the topical administration of a solution of 2.5% methacholine
(4) In sympathetic denervation, the pupil will dilate upon the topical administration of cocaine

460. Correct statements concerning multiple sclerosis include which of the following?

(1) Optic neuritis is a presenting manifestation in 25 percent of patients
(2) Seizures occur in approximately 40 percent of patients over the course of the disease
(3) Cerebellar ataxia may be found combined with sensory ataxia
(4) Peripheral nerve involvement with absent reflexes may occur

461. In older people, amyotrophic lateral sclerosis and cervical spondylosis may mimic each other. Laboratory tests that help to distinguish these disorders include

(1) nerve conduction velocity measurements
(2) electromyography
(3) cerebrospinal fluid protein electrophoresis
(4) myelography

DIRECTIONS: Each group of questions below consists of lettered headings followed by a set of numbered items. For each numbered item select the **one** lettered heading with which it is **most** closely associated. Each lettered heading may be used **once, more than once, or not at all.**

Questions 462–466

Match each description to the appropriate tumor.

(A) Meningioma
(B) Astrocytoma
(C) Glioblastoma multiforme
(D) Hemangioblastoma
(E) Medulloblastoma

462. Tendency to form large cavities; between 60 and 75 percent of patients have recurrent seizures; slowly growing

463. Sharply demarcated from brain tissue; psammoma bodies present microscopically; highest incidence in seventh decade

464. Frequently fills the fourth ventricle; majority of patients are children 4 to 8 years of age; stumbling gait, frequent falls, and papilledema found on presentation

465. Accounts for 20 percent of all intracranial tumors; 50 percent are bilateral; may form distant foci on spinal roots; seizures present in 30 to 40 percent of patients

466. Presents with dizziness, ataxia of gait, and symptoms and signs of increased intracranial pressure; polycythemia; displays dominant inheritance

Questions 467–470

Match the descriptions below with the appropriate disorder.

(A) Temporal arteritis
(B) Polyarteritis nodosa
(C) Systemic lupus erythematosus
(D) Takayasu's disease
(E) None of the above

467. Seizures, mental status changes, and cranial nerve findings are common neurologic manifestations

468. Constitutional symptoms are prominent; occlusion of subclavian and carotid arteries is typical

469. CNS involvement is rare; may give rise to a symmetric polyneuropathy

470. Significant inflammation of intracranial arteries is rare; affects large and medium arteries; occurs commonly in elderly persons

Questions 471–474

For each of the complexes of neurologic findings below, select the disorder with which it is most closely related.

(A) Poliomyelitis
(B) Amyotrophic lateral sclerosis
(C) Pernicious anemia
(D) Multiple sclerosis
(E) Cervical spondylosis

471. Asymmetric motor, sensory, and bladder symptoms, each developing at a different time

472. Asymmetric muscle atrophy and loss of deep tendon reflexes in one leg

473. Spasticity and loss of vibration in the legs, with radicular pain and muscle atrophy in the arms

474. Fairly symmetric muscle atrophy and hyperreflexia of the arms and legs, with sensory function intact

DIRECTIONS: The group of questions below consists of four lettered headings followed by a set of numbered items. For each numbered item select

A	if the item is associated with	(A) **only**
B	if the item is associated with	(B) **only**
C	if the item is associated with	**both** (A) and (B)
D	if the item is associated with	**neither** (A) nor (B)

Each lettered heading may be used **once, more than once, or not at all.**

Questions 475–478

    (A) Botulism
    (B) Guillain-Barré syndrome
    (C) Both
    (D) Neither

475. Cranial nerve involvement

476. Response to edrophonium

477. Fever

478. Ascending paralysis

Neurology
Answers

439.   The answer is E. *(Braunwald, ed 11. pp 2082–2084.)* Periodic paralysis may develop from inherited or acquired conditions that cause acute changes in the level of serum potassium. A rapid flow of potassium from the serum into muscles changes the muscle membrane potential, making muscle fibers electrically inexcitable until the potassium defect is corrected. Three hereditary forms of this problem can be recognized. In one, which usually comes on during the second decade of life, serum potassium levels fall during an attack to less than 3 mEq/L. Often these attacks are brought on by large meals or strenuous exercise. The hypokalemia can be so severe that ECG changes of hypokalemia are detectable. A second form of the condition occurs at a young age, and the serum potassium level remains normal during attacks. Emotional stress, exercise, and alcohol can bring on this form of the disease, which produces chronic attacks that may last up to 2 weeks. A third form involves the elevation of serum potassium during an attack to levels in excess of 5.5 mEq/L. Again, exercise may precipitate paralysis, but so will the administration of potassium or exposure to cold. In this condition paralysis is often localized to the muscles of the tongue and eyelids. Periodic paralysis may also develop when hypokalemia is secondary to a loss of the electrolyte through the kidney or intestinal tract. Excessive licorice ingestion or thyrotoxicosis may also produce the same effect. Whereas in the latter cases treatment is directed toward the basic defect causing the problem, the hereditary form of the disease can often be managed well by the administration of acetazolamide. In cases of hypokalemic paralysis the drug induces an acidosis that is thought to protect the patient from paralysis by blocking potassium shifts from serum to muscle. In the hyperkalemic paralysis the drug is thought to promote the loss of potassium through the urine. Although it is unusual for attacks to be fatal, it may well be that this patient's father, while driving, developed weakness that impaired his skills and led to his fatal accident.

440.   The answer is D. *(Adams, ed 3. pp 49, 1010. Braunwald, ed 11. pp 82–83, 1947–1949.)* The diabetic patient described in the question has weakness of one side of a cranial structure, in this instance the face, and weakness of the opposite side of the body, in this instance the right arm and leg. This "crossed hemiplegia" is characteristic of brainstem lesions. The cranial nerve nuclei, of course, are ipsilateral to the structures that their nerves innervate; in this patient, it is the left sixth and seventh cranial nerves that are affected. However, because her lesion is *above* the level of decussation of the pyramidal tract, the arm and leg *contralateral* to the lesion site are affected.

441. The answer is C. *(Wilson, ed 7. p 728.)* Delayed relaxation of tendon reflexes is a strong physical finding favoring a diagnosis of hypothyroidism. It is believed to be due not to any neurologic pathology but to a slowing of muscular contraction and relaxation. While precise measurement of the reflex may be accomplished by using a photomotogram, its utility is limited by the fact that fully one-third of hypothyroid patients have values within the normal range. Furthermore, the delay in reflex relaxation occurs in nonthyroid conditions as well, including anorexia nervosa, peripheral vascular disease, edematous states, and propranolol and procainamide administration, in addition to the conditions listed in the question (with the exception of Addison's disease).

442. The answer is D. *(Mandell, ed 2. pp 585–591.)* Brain abscess is a focal suppurative cerebral inflammatory process with a mortality of 15 to 20 percent. Predisposing factors include a contiguous source of infection, cyanotic congenital heart disease, trauma, and chronic pyogenic lung diseases. Common microbiologic isolates of abscesses are *Staphylococcus aureus* (especially after trauma), Enterobacteriaceae members, streptococci, and fungi in patients who are immunocompromised. Solitary brain abscess occurs most commonly in the frontal and temporal lobes. The classic triad of fever, headache, and focal neurologic defect is found in a minority of patients; indeed, fully 50 to 55 percent of patients may be afebrile and only half may have a focal defect. The diagnosis should be considered, then, in any patient with neurologic findings and a predisposing factor to cerebral abscess. Because CSF findings are nonspecific and the risk of herniation is significant, lumbar puncture is contraindicated and CT scanning remains the diagnostic procedure of choice. Treatment involves long-term antibiotic administration and most patients require surgical drainage for optimal management.

443. The answer is C. *(Braunwald, ed 11. pp 40–41, 2067–2068.)* Local weakness involving one or both arms that frequently starts off as severe pain and progresses to weakness as the pain abates may signal the onset of a brachial plexus neuropathy. Although this syndrome can develop without any precipitating cause being recognized, it is not uncommon for it to follow immunization or antitoxin administration. The fact that viral infection (especially influenza) precedes the paralysis makes it likely that an immunological reaction is involved. Young men are affected more commonly, and it is not unusual to find a familial incidence of the problem. The upper part of the brachial plexus is most commonly involved, and thus the maximum weakness will be found in the shoulder girdle. Sensory loss is usually minimal. Nerve conduction studies may identify a local disturbance and myelography is not necessary in this condition. The prognosis is excellent and no specific treatment is required, though patients must be warned that sometimes it may take up to 2 years for a full return to normal function.

444. The answer is D. *(Braunwald, ed 11. pp 2017–2019. Lees, J Neurol Neurosurg Psychiatry 44:1020, 1981.)* Nerve fibers from the substantia nigra pass into the corpus striatum with a release of the potent neurotransmitter dopamine. In Parkinson's disease degenerative changes occur in the substantia nigra, particularly in that subsegment known as the pars compacta. The result is a loss of the neurotransmitter dopamine, a biochemical defect that produces the syndrome known as Parkinson's disease, or paralysis agitans. The incidence of this disease has been stated in various series to range from 60 to 200 per 100,000 population. The disease is twice as common in men as in women and a family history is not unusual. Therapy for Parkinson's disease is designed to provide dopamine for the central nervous system. As dopamine itself will not cross the blood-brain barrier the mainstay of therapy is levodopa, which is a precursor for dopamine synthesis that can cross the blood-brain barrier and reach the basal ganglia. The drug is usually administered in combination with carbidopa. The latter agent prevents levodopa from being converted to dopamine in peripheral tissues. As carbidopa does not cross the blood-brain barrier, it will not interfere with the formation of dopamine from levodopa in the central nervous system. Because of the severe side effects that are associated with the long-term administration of levodopa, especially as the disease worsens, many physicians try to avoid therapy with this agent until it is absolutely necessary. Amantadine is an agent that stimulates the release of dopamine stored at nerve terminals in the brain and is successful in managing the tremor, particularly in the earlier stages of the disease. Once patients have started on levodopa, the regimen they require will need individual tailoring. Some need different doses depending on the time of day and the physical activity they are planning. There are major side effects from the administration of levodopa, and these must constantly be sought. Cardiac arrhythmias, gastrointestinal hemorrhage, and psychiatric disturbances occur in 30 percent of patients on chronic therapy. Dyskinesia develops in approximately 80 percent of patients who receive the drug for more than 1 year. This takes the form of involuntary movement that can be mild or very severe. Involuntary movements may eventually become quite disabling. Sometimes the dyskinesia gives way to akinesia with frozen postural attitudes, fixed facies being characteristic. In an attempt to limit the amount of levodopa that must be given to patients, combination therapy is often tried. One recently successful approach has been to use the drug bromocriptine, which acts as an agonist for the dopamine receptor in the brain. As it can directly stimulate this receptor, the advantages for patients who are no longer responding well to levodopa are obvious. As neuronal degeneration progresses in Parkinson's disease, the biochemical mechanisms needed to convert levodopa to dopamine fail. Refractoriness to levodopa will therefore develop.

445. The answer is E. *(Adams, ed 3. pp 834–835. Braunwald, ed 11. pp 119–120.)* Patients in coma following drug intoxication have a fairly good chance of full recovery, provided they are still breathing by the time help is available. Extreme hypothermia, especially in combination with a mild intoxication, may also provide a comatose condition that is reversible. No other causes for coma have been associated with a reasonable chance of full recovery.

446. The answer is E. *(Braunwald, ed 11. pp 29–33. Lance, Ann Neurol 10:1, 1981.)* A number of conditions that produce headaches may mimic migraine. In attempting to work up a differential diagnosis, therefore, the physician should keep in mind that migraine is characteristically a disorder that starts in youth and that headaches that come on in middle age are probably due to some other problem. Although it is common for patients to have neurological symptoms and signs as a migraine headache develops and during the course of the pain, it is unusual for the symptoms to persist once the headache departs. Persistence of a visual field defect or speech disturbance or even a mild hemiparesis suggests a focal lesion. Similarly, involvement of the first division of the trigeminal nerve producing a loss of sensation on the face when associated with headache strongly suggests that a lesion exists near the cavernous sinus and a CT scan is indicated. Periodic headache due to the raising of intracranial pressure may be precipitated by coughing, sneezing, or even bending over. Many patients whose headaches are triggered in this fashion have brain tumors. There are a number of conditions that do precipitate genuine migraine headaches, however. These include an excess amount of sleep, a change in the weather, irregular hours, a change in eating habits (such as missing a meal), the consumption of alcohol, menstruation, and the ingestion of birth control pills. Of interest, migraine headaches usually disappear in women who are pregnant only to frequently return with more severity in the immediate postpartum period.

447. The answer is E. *(Braunwald, ed 11. pp 41, 386, 2024–2026, 2045–2046.)* Vitamin B_{12} deficiency, apart from producing pernicious anemia, affects the nervous system, characteristically producing a subacute combined degeneration of the spinal cord, involving posterior column and pyramidal tract lesions. Peripheral neuropathy occurs in addition. Multiple disc lesions, particularly those that occur at the L5-S1 region in combination with defects above this level, may cause a myelopathy. Progressive degeneration of unknown etiology of motor neurons may occur in the cerebral cortex, brainstem, and spinal cord, or in any combination thereof. Such degeneration usually is grouped under the heading of motor neuron disease or motor system disease. Depending on the areas of the nervous system predominantly involved, subdivisions can be recognized. The most commonly occurring form of motor system disease, associated with muscular atrophy and hyperreflexia, is amyotrophic lateral sclerosis. A progressive muscular atrophy and progressive bulbar palsy, together with primary lateral sclerosis, can also present a distinctive syndrome. Both motor system disease and syringomyelia may give rise to upper motor neuron lesions and to a lower motor neuron lesion at the L5-S1 nerve root, thus producing the upper motor neuron sign of extensor plantar reflexes and the lower motor neuron sign of absent ankle reflexes. A tumor of the cauda equina, which occurs below the end of the upper motor neurons, thus cannot produce extensor plantar reflexes.

448. The answer is C. *(Braunwald, ed 11. pp 2000–2003.)* Wernicke's disease, as exemplified in the patient presented in the question, is characterized by ocular disturbances consisting of (1) weakness or paralysis of external recti, (2) nystagmus, and (3) various paralyses of conjugate gaze. Ataxia and a global confusion state also are characteristic. In more than 80 percent of affected patients, polyneuropathy occurs. Korsakoff's psychosis, known also as the amnesia-confabulatory syndrome, is not a separate disease but a variably present psychic component of Wernicke's disease involving impairment of retentive memory and learning ability. When both neurological and psychic elements of the disease are present, it is known as the Wernicke-Korsakoff syndrome. Marchiafava-Bignami disease, which is seen chiefly in Italian men who are heavy wine drinkers, is associated with bilateral demyelinization of the corpus callosum; clinically, this disease is characterized by (1) emotional disorders, (2) loss of mental faculties, (3) convulsions, and (4) a variety of motor disabilities.

449. The answer is B. *(Braunwald, ed 11. p 846.)* Methanol is a component of antifreeze and, because of its inebriating property, may be used by the indigent alcoholic. It is oxidized relatively slowly by alcohol dehydrogenase to formaldehyde and then to formic acid, which causes the resultant acidosis and retinal damage. Symptoms of methanol poisoning typically appear 12 to 24 hours after ingestion and include headache, nausea and vomiting, dizziness, and visual disturbances. The pupils become dilated and unreactive and permanent blindness may occur with as little as 15 ml of methanol. Treatment involves correction of the acidosis, infusion of alcohol to competitively inhibit the metabolism of methanol, and hemodialysis when methanol blood levels exceed 50 mg/dl.

450. The answer is E (all). *(Adams, ed 3. pp 294–296. Braunwald, ed 11. pp 112–113.)* Patients with narcolepsy usually present complaining of excessive sleepiness during the daytime. Frequently uncontrollable drowsiness will come over them, often lasting for periods of up to 15 minutes. At the end of this time patients awake feeling fully refreshed. Obviously the disease causes considerable embarrassment and can put patients into an extremely dangerous situation if they happen to be driving a car or carrying out some dangerous occupation when an attack strikes. Although boring situations can precipitate an attack for victims of this disease, it is common for an intensely emotional or exciting experience to be the cause. Some variations of the narcoleptic syndrome have been described. Some patients, particularly after an emotional experience such as intense laughing, will develop a sudden paralysis of their lower limbs. Others, when they are coming out of a period of sleep, will experience a transient quadraplegia or terrifying hallucinations. There is evidence to suggest that a basic defect in sleep regulation exists in these patients. Characteristically, normal persons on falling asleep will have 1 to 2 hours of non-REM sleep before they enter their first REM period. During the night they will then alternate between non-REM and REM periods. It is during REM periods that dreaming occurs and the movement of muscles is inhibited. Patients with narcolepsy slip immediately into REM sleep patterns and these are prolonged. Numerous stimulants have been tried in patients with narcolepsy. The drug of choice is methylphenidate, 5 to 10 mg by mouth three times a day. For those patients who experience sensations of paralysis associated with their narcolepsy, imipramine, 25 mg by mouth three times a day, can often be added with success. It is obviously important for a physician to discuss the lifestyle of his patients so that together they can work out strategies for handling potentially dangerous situations. Patients should, of course, be warned not to drive until attacks are under control.

451. The answer is E (all). *(Adams, ed 3. pp 1034–1037, 1044–1056.)* Polymyositis is characterized by a symmetric weakness of proximal limb and trunk muscles and is associated with other connective tissue diseases in up to one-half of cases. In the majority of patients, serum CK and aldolase levels are markedly increased and myoglobinuria is typically present. EMG analysis reveals many fibrillation potentials and pseudomyotonic activity. Biopsy of affected tissue shows marked regeneration and degeneration of muscle. Clinically, muscle weakness may proceed rapidly over a period of several weeks to months. Treatment with prednisone is beneficial in most patients; those who are refractory may respond to methotrexate or azathioprine. The muscular dystrophies are hereditary degenerative diseases of skeletal muscle that also cause a symmetric muscular weakness. In contrast to polymyositis, they generally evolve over a longer period of time; muscle enzyme levels are not as high, although the Duchenne type of dystrophy, a disease of children, is associated with high levels of CK and aldolase; and no treatment is currently available. EMG is characterized by small action potentials during partial and full voluntary contraction. Biopsy of affected tissue reveals loss of muscle fibers, segmental necrosis, regenerative activity, fibrosis, and an increase in lipocytes.

452. The answer is A (1, 2, 3). *(Adams, ed 3. pp 599–604.)* TIAs are due to atherosclerotic vascular disease and are reversible neurologic deficits that last no more than 24 hours. In one study, the 5-year cumulative rate of cerebral infarction was 22.7 percent and, for those with carotid lesions, the rate of myocardial infarction was 21 percent. There are no characteristics that distinguish those patients with TIAs who will go on to stroke from those who will not. TIAs of the carotid system typically result in either ipsilateral monocular blindness or contralateral sensorimotor disturbances; they do not occur simultaneously. TIAs of the vertebral-basilar system are characterized by dysarthria, bifacial numbness, staggering, blindness, headache, and nausea and vomiting. While controversial, antiplatelet drugs seem to reduce the risk of stroke and death; the role of surgical therapy is controversial, as well.

453. The answer is C (2, 4). *(Adams, ed 3. p 657.)* Epilepsy occurs in 5 percent of patients with closed-head injuries and only in those who sustain a contusion or laceration of the cortex. The seizures are either focal or generalized and only rarely are they of the petit mal variety. The timing of posttrauma seizures varies; approximately half of patients who will develop epilepsy will have their first attack within

6 months of injury. They tend to decrease in frequency with time and up to 30 percent of patients will stop having them. Patients who have their first attack within a week of injury are more likely to have a complete remission than those patients whose first attack occurs over a year after trauma.

454. The answer is B (1, 3). *(Adams, ed 3. pp 468–469.)* Pseudotumor cerebri is a syndrome of unknown origin characterized by extreme elevations of CSF pressure, typically to 250 to 450 mm H_2O. Patients present complaining of headache, blurred vision, and dizziness, while the neurologic examination is remarkable only for papilledema and, rarely, for an abducens palsy or nystagmus. Visual field testing shows enlargement of the blind spots along with peripheral constriction. The only severe consequence of this entity is blindness in those patients who do not respond to either repeated lumbar punctures or lumbar thecoperitoneal shunting. Therapy with steroids or oral hyperosmotic agents is of controversial benefit.

455. The answer is A (1, 2, 3). *(Adams, ed 3. pp 869–872.)* Huntington's chorea is an autosomal dominant disorder characterized by choreoathetosis and dementia. It is believed to be due, at least in part, to an increased sensitivity of striatal receptors to dopamine and to a decrease in the enzymes glutamic acid decarboxylase and choline acetyltransferase in the striatum and lateral pallidum. Pathologically, a bilateral wasting of the head of the caudate nucleus and putamen is seen. Patients present with disturbances in mood, poor self-control, changes in personality, a gradual fall in intellect, and choreoathetosis; the movement disorder and mental symptoms may present at any time in relation to each other. Symptoms may be alleviated somewhat with the use of phenothiazines and butyrophenones. Huntington's chorea runs a progressive course, however, with death occurring an average of 15 years after onset.

456. The answer is E (all). *(Braunwald, ed 11. pp 1729–1731.)* SIADH is characterized by an inappropriate release of antidiuretic hormone resulting in hyponatremia in the presence of a urine hypertonic relative to plasma. The pathogenesis of SIADH is categorized under malignancy, pulmonary disease, CNS dysfunction, drugs, and miscellaneous causes such as hypothyroidism and positive pressure ventilation. CNS causes other than those listed in the question include skull fracture, subdural hematoma, cerebral atrophy, SLE, and acute intermittent porphyria. SIADH due to these causes results from inappropriate neurohypophyseal release of ADH in response to the surrounding pathologic stimulus.

457. The answer is A (1, 2, 3). *(Adams, ed 3. pp 625–626.)* Hypertensive encephalopathy is a syndrome characterized by diffuse cerebral disturbance that occurs as a result of an elevated blood pressure. Symptoms typically include headache, nausea and vomiting, convulsions, and visual disturbances; focal neurologic signs may occur but suggest an associated structural lesion. While encephalopathy may be a complication of hypertension due to any cause, it is more common in patients with essential hypertension and seems to be more common in blacks. Diagnosis is made on clinical grounds, although the CSF abnormalities of elevated pressure and protein, while nonspecific, are present in almost all cases. Symptoms are reversed within 72 hours of appropriate therapy.

458. The answer is E (all). *(Braunwald, ed 11. pp 1349–1350, 2007–2008.)* Hepatic encephalopathy is a neuropsychiatric disorder occurring in patients with hepatocellular disease or in those with portal-systemic venous shunting. It is characterized by asterixis; alterations of personality and mentation, which may progress to stupor and coma; and generalized slowing of cerebral electrical activity accompanied by high voltage and slow-wave forms on EEG. It is thought to be secondary to the accumulation of toxic metabolites, such as ammonia, that are normally cleared by the liver. Increased protein intake and gastrointestinal bleeding, both of which cause colonic bacteria to produce more ammonia, and alkalosis, which allows for a greater concentration of uncharged ammonia to cross the blood-brain barrier, are common precipitants of hepatic encephalopathy. In addition to ammonia, glutamine, α-ketoglutarate, tryptophan, mercaptan, short-chain fatty acids, infection, altered permeability of the blood-brain barrier, and other factors have been implicated in its pathogenesis.

459. The answer is B (1, 3). *(Adams, ed 3. p 403.)* In the pharmacologic evaluation of pupillary innervation, it is helpful to remember the concept of a denervation hypersensitivity, a phenomenon in which an effector organ becomes hypersensitive to its particular neurotransmitter, and to related drugs, 2 to 3 weeks after denervation. The topical administration of a 1:1000 solution of epinephrine has no effect on the normal pupil but will dilate the sympathetically denervated pupil, a result seen to a greater degree with lesions of postganglionic fibers than of preganglionic fibers. Contrariwise, the pupil rarely reacts with lesions involving central sympathetic pathways. Cocaine prevents the reuptake of epinephrine into nerve endings and thereby potentiates the effect of the transmitter; the normal eye dilates while no effect on pupillary size is seen with sympathetic denervation. The normal pupil does not respond to the topical administration of a 2.5% solution of methacholine, while the denervated pupil will constrict.

460. The answer is B (1, 3). *(Adams, ed 3. pp 703–707. Braunwald, ed 11. pp 1995–1997.)* Multiple sclerosis is a chronic neurological disease characterized by recurrent episodes—over a period of 20 to 30 years—of optic neuritis and symptoms due to brainstem and spinal cord involvement. Seizures, however, occur in only about 5 percent of affected patients. In multiple sclerosis, the central nervous system is always involved and the peripheral nerves are not. The disease is rarely found between latitudes 35° north and south. Persons who migrate from high-risk to low-risk areas retain their susceptibility to multiple sclerosis. Of the many manifestations of the disease, cerebellar ataxia, often very severe, may coexist with sensory ataxia due to involvement of the posterior columns of the spinal cord.

461. The answer is C (2, 4). *(Adams, ed 3. pp 687, 709. Braunwald, ed 11. pp 2024–2025, 2044–2045.)* The tests commonly employed to help distinguish amyotrophic lateral sclerosis (ALS) from cervical spondylosis are electromyography and myelography. Electromyography may disclose involvement of anterior horn cells outside the cervical region, thus favoring the diagnosis of ALS. Myelography may demonstrate a compressive lesion of the cervical spinal cord, thus pointing to cervical spondylosis.

462–466. The answers are: 462-B, 463-A, 464-E, 465-C, 466-D. *(Adams, ed 3. pp 482–493.)* Glioblastoma multiforme accounts for 20 percent of all intracranial tumors and is highly malignant. While predominantly cerebral in location, tumors may be found in the cerebellum, brainstem, or spinal cord. Malignant cells may form distant foci on spinal roots or cause a meningeal gliomatosis; extraneural metastases are very rare. About 50 percent are bilateral and between 3 and 6 percent show multicentric foci of growth. The prognosis is poor as less than a fifth of all patients survive for 1 year after onset of symptoms.

An astrocytoma may occur anywhere in the brain or spinal cord. It is slowly growing and infiltrative and has a tendency to form pseudocysts. Calcium may be deposited in part of the tumor. Half of patients present with focal seizures; the onset of focal seizures in persons 20 to 60 years of age should raise the suspicion of an astrocytoma. In cases of cerebral astrocytoma, the average survival after the first symptom is 5 years; for cerebellar tumors, it is 7 years.

A meningioma is a benign tumor that is always sharply demarcated from brain tissue and is slowly growing. The most common sites are the Sylvian region, superior parasagittal surface of frontal and parietal lobes, olfactory grooves, lesser wings of the sphenoid bones, tuberculum sellae, superior surface of the cerebellum, cerebellopontine angles, and spinal canal. Surgical excision affords a permanent cure.

Medulloblastoma, primarily a childhood tumor, arises in the posterior part of the cerebellar vermis and neuroepithelial roof of the fourth ventricle. It is well demarcated from the adjacent brain tissue. Typically, patients present complaining of repeated vomiting and a morning headache, followed by a stumbling gait, frequent falls, and a squint. Therapy with surgery, radiation of the neuraxis, and chemotherapy yields a 5-year survival in more than two-thirds of cases.

Hemangioblastoma of the cerebellum is characterized by dizziness, ataxia of gait, signs and symptoms of increased intracranial pressure, and, in some cases, an associated retinal angioma. Polycythemia may result from elaboration of an erythropoietic factor from the tumor.

467–470. The answers are: 467-C, 468-D, 469-B, 470-A. *(Adams, ed 3. pp 626–629.)* Nonbacterial inflammatory diseases that involve cranial arteries are a diverse group of disorders with varied clinical consequences. Temporal arteritis is an inflammation of large and medium arteries and principally afflicts the elderly. Constitutional symptoms frequently precede symptoms of arterial involvement. Arteritis of the temporal artery manifests as headache and may lead to blindness in 25 percent of patients. Commonly, the arteritis involves the aorta and its major branches and leads to ischemia and infarction of involved body sites. Treatment with prednisone arrests the disease.

Polyarteritis nodosa is a widespread inflammation of medium and small arteries with only rare pulmonary involvement. Along with constitutional symptoms, patients frequently complain of muscle weakness, arthralgias, and abdominal symptoms. The arteritis may cause digital gangrene, renal failure, coronary ischemia, and, because it involves the vasa nervorum, mononeuritis multiplex or a symmetric polyneuropathy.

SLE is a multisystem disease characterized by antibodies to nuclear components. Neurologic disorders occur in 20 to 50 percent of patients and common manifestations include seizures, mental status changes, cranial nerve involvement, and transverse myelitis; peripheral neuropathies are infrequent. The pathogenesis of most of the neurologic disease seen in SLE seems to involve multiple cortical and brainstem microinfarcts.

Takayasu's disease is a nonspecific arteritis of the aorta and the major arteries of the aortic arch; it typically affects young Asian women. Initially, constitutional symptoms are prominent; there then follows a stage dominated by the consequences of stenosis or occlusion of major arteries. Syncope, blurred vision, paresthesias, claudication, and hypertension are common presenting features and reflect involvement of the carotid, vertebral, subclavian, and renal arteries. There is currently no effective treatment; death occurs within 5 years of diagnosis.

471–474. The answers are: 471-D, 472-A, 473-E, 474-B. *(Adams, ed 3. pp 171, 547–551, 700–711, 773–776, 889–890, 892. Braunwald, ed 11. pp 705, 1995–1997, 2024–2025, 2044–2045.)* Multiple sclerosis produces a combination of motor, sensory, bladder, and cranial nerve symptoms. They usually occur asymmetrically, affecting different parts of the central nervous system with each attack. The less common, slowly progressive form of the disease also affects different structures at different times.

Poliomyelitis produces asymmetric muscle atrophy and loss of deep tendon reflexes, sometimes confined to one limb. The feature of polio that would separate it from a neuropathy or radiculopathy is the complete absence of sensory loss. While amyotrophic lateral sclerosis also may produce asymmetric muscle atrophy and loss of some deep tendon reflexes, hyperreflexia commonly exists in this disease, and it usually involves more than one limb.

Cervical spondylosis is a condition in which both cervical root compression and spinal cord compression may occur. The spinal cord compression will produce long tract signs including spasticity and loss of vibration sense in the legs. The root compression in the neck will produce radicular pain and muscle atrophy in the arms.

Amyotrophic lateral sclerosis, a degeneration of anterior horn cells, results in muscle atrophy that may be fairly symmetric. There also is degeneration of cortical neurons in the motor areas, along with their descending tracts—a process that produces hyperreflexia. The sensory findings should be essentially normal in patients who have amyotrophic lateral sclerosis.

475–478. The answers are: 475-C, 476-A, 477-D, 478-B. *(Mandell, ed 2. pp 1360–1362. Sunderrajan, Medicine 64:333–341, 1985.)* The Guillain-Barré syndrome is an acute polyneuropathy that may present as an ascending motor paralysis, ophthalmoplegia with ataxia and areflexia, or a painful, sensory polyneuritis. The major manifestation is symmetrical weakness affecting the proximal and distal muscles in an ascending fashion, although occasionally cranial and upper extremity muscles are affected first. In the vast majority of patients, the cerebrospinal fluid is completely normal.

Botulism, in contrast, is a symmetric descending paralysis caused by neurotoxins elaborated by *Clostridium botulinum* obtained through food poisoning or trauma. The toxins produce their clinical effects by preventing acetylcholine release from peripheral cholinergic synapses. Fatigue, dry mouth, constipation, postural hypotension, urinary retention, and muscular weakness are common complications. Typically, cranial nerves are affected first, followed by a descending paralysis that involves the respiratory musculature, as well. Deep tendon reflexes are variably affected. Interestingly, a few patients with botulism respond to edrophonium, although not to the degree seen in myasthenia gravis. Treatment involves the use of antitoxin and intensive respiratory therapy; recovery is gradual over weeks to months.

Dermatology

DIRECTIONS: Each question below contains five suggested responses. Select the **one best** response to each question.

479. A patient receiving thiazide diuretics or sulfonamides who is subject to photosensitive drug reactions may use all the following sunscreens EXCEPT

(A) benzophenones
(B) zinc oxide
(C) titanium oxide
(D) kaolin
(E) para-aminobenzoic acid (PABA)

480. A 20-year-old woman is complaining of several days of low-grade fever, malaise, and mild conjunctivitis. Soon after the onset of fever, she developed a rash along with swelling of the joints of fingers, wrists, and knees in a symmetric fashion. The rash consists of discrete pink macules, which began on her face and extended to her trunk. She is also noted to have small red spots on her palate. Her arthritis is a complication of which of the following?

(A) Toxic shock syndrome
(B) Porphyria cutanea tarda
(C) Reiter's syndrome
(D) Rubella
(E) Gonococcal bacteremia

481. Exfoliative dermatitis is characterized by all the following statements EXCEPT that it

(A) can occur as a result of a preexisting dermatitis
(B) occurs in association with lymphoma
(C) may involve all the skin surface
(D) is a scaling, erythematous lesion
(E) is associated with a 10 percent mortality

482. Psoralens, of which methoxsalen is an example, are effective in all the following diseases EXCEPT

(A) psoriasis
(B) vitiligo
(C) eczema
(D) mycosis fungoides
(E) porphyria cutanea tarda

483. Pyoderma gangrenosum is associated with all the following EXCEPT

(A) inflammatory bowel disease
(B) Wegener's granulomatosis
(C) primary biliary cirrhosis
(D) trauma
(E) paraproteinemia

484. A 78-year-old derelict man is hospitalized for an acute myocardial infarction. On physical examination, he is found to have coiled hairs and petechial rash distributed around the hair follicles. These abnormalities are most obvious in the groin and thighs. The patient's gums are bloody. The most probable cause of this man's skin lesions is

(A) leukemia cutis
(B) thrombocytopenia
(C) kwashiorkor
✓(D) vitamin C deficiency
(E) niacin deficiency

485. All the following statements about aphthous stomatitis (canker sores) are correct EXCEPT

(A) the lesions occur singly or in groups and usually heal in 10 to 14 days
(B) the tendency to develop aphthous ulceration is linked to the expression of the HLA antigens A2 and B12
✗(C) Coxsackie virus is frequently cultured from the lesions
(D) aphthous stomatitis can be associated with Crohn's disease
(E) at least 20 percent of the general population suffer the pain and discomfort of these outbreaks

486. Generalized exfoliative dermatitis is caused by which of the following disorders?

(A) Erythema multiforme
(B) Pemphigus vulgaris
✓(C) Mycosis fungoides
(D) Angiokeratoma corporis diffusum
(E) Atrophoderma of Pasini and Pierini

487. A 39-year-old woman has had nonhealing painful erosions in her mouth for the past year. She now observes rapidly spreading blisters on her chest and erosions of her scalp; the lesions are flaccid and red at the base. A biopsy report notes acantholysis of the prickle cells and deposition of IgG and complement in the intercellular spaces of the epidermis. Which of the following statements best summarizes both this woman's disorder and the appropriate treatment?

(A) She has a blistering disorder and should be treated with the most potent topical steroids, e.g., 0.5% triamcinolone (Aristocort) applied every 2 to 3 hours
(B) She has an autoimmune disorder and should be treated with 6-mercaptopurine or methotrexate
✓(C) She has a disease that is fatal unless treated with prednisone, 100 mg or more daily
(D) She has cutaneous lupus erythematosus and should receive oral hydroxychloroquine, 400 mg a day
(E) She has bullous impetigo and needs oral penicillinase-resistant antibiotics for 7 to 10 days

488. Herpes zoster (shingles) is characterized by all the following statements EXCEPT that it

(A) is caused by varicella virus
(B) typically produces a few scattered vesicles
✗(C) has a high rate of recurrence
(D) is not contagious for people who have had chickenpox
(E) has a significant association with malignant lymphoma

489. Diabetes mellitus is associated with all the following cutaneous signs EXCEPT

(A) granuloma annulare
(B) necrobiosis lipoidica
(C) lipoatrophy
(D) brown atrophic macules on the pretibial surface
X (E) lichen simplex chronicus

490. An asymptomatic 20-year-old man is noted to have a 4-cm lesion on his back that appeared approximately 10 years ago as a brown patch. Over the years, the lesion developed a growth of coarse and darkly pigmented hair. Which of the following is the likely diagnosis?

(A) Café au lait macule
✓ (B) Becker's nevus
(C) Nevus sebaceous
(D) Epidermal nevus
(E) Mongolian spot

491. A young woman has recurrent episodes, lasting 1 to 2 weeks, of very painful ulcers scattered over the labial and buccal mucosa and occasionally on the pharynx. No blisters appear. Her lesions have no apparent association with stress, fever, or menses. The oval ulcers are 1 to 2 mm in size with a gray base and red border. The most likely diagnosis is

(A) herpes simplex
(B) herpes zoster
✓ (C) aphthous stomatitis
(D) contact dermatitis
(E) desquamative gingivitis

492. Psoriasis is characterized by all the following statements EXCEPT that

(A) it affects more than 2 percent of the population
X (B) lesions rarely occur on the scalp
(C) it consists of isolated scaling papules or plaques
(D) the borders of the plaques are distinct
(E) the plaques are pink to deep red

493. A 28-year-old woman who is 3 months post partum notes a distressing loss of scalp hair. A meticulous physical examination is unremarkable; the scalp and hair appear normal, and there are no bald spots. The patient takes no medications and says that she feels well. The most likely cause of hair loss is

(A) postpartum hypothyroidism
✓ (B) postpartum telogen effluvium
(C) hypervitaminosis due to vitamin supplementation during pregnancy
(D) trichotillomania
(E) alopecia areata

494. Generalized pruritus without diagnostic skin lesions occurs in all the following conditions EXCEPT

(A) hyperthyroidism
(B) polycythemia vera
(C) carcinoid syndrome
X (D) secondary syphilis
(E) pregnancy

DIRECTIONS: The questions below contain four suggested responses of which **one or more** is correct. Select

A	if	**1, 2, and 3**	are correct
B	if	**1 and 3**	are correct
C	if	**2 and 4**	are correct
D	if	**4**	is correct
E	if	**1, 2, 3, and 4**	are correct

495. A 28-year-old homosexual man is noted to have several purplish macules located on the soles of both feet. Biopsy of a typical lesion reveals a mixture of spindle cells and endothelial cells with bands of fibrous tissue. This lesion is characterized by which of the following statements?

(1) Mucosal involvement is rare
(2) Brain metastases are uncommon
(3) It generally follows an indolent course
(4) It is radiosensitive

496. Cutaneous manifestations shared by variegate porphyria and porphyria cutanea tarda include

(1) hypertrichosis
(2) bullous lesions
(3) depigmented scars
(4) facial hyperpigmentation

497. Idiopathic skin signs of internal malignancy include

(1) migratory thrombophlebitis
(2) ichthyosis
(3) hypertrichosis lanugosa
(4) pachydermoperiostosis

498. Nail pitting is associated with which of the following skin diseases?

(1) Scleroderma
(2) Psoriasis
(3) Lichen planus
(4) Alopecia areata

499. A 55-year-old man with a history of rheumatoid arthritis treated with an arsenical compound many years ago is now noted to have a lesion on the volar aspect of his right arm. It is a sharply demarcated, hyperkeratotic, fissured, brownish-red plaque that has extended gradually over the past few years. Which of the following should be included in this man's therapy?

(1) Surgical excision of the lesion
(2) Systemic chemotherapy
(3) Examinations to detect visceral neoplasia
(4) Psoralen photochemotherapy (PUVA)

500. Lesions associated with Reiter's syndrome include

(1) painless oral ulcers
(2) circinate balanitis
(3) keratoderma blenorrhagica
(4) granuloma annulare

Dermatology

Answers

479. The answer is E. *(Braunwald, ed 11. p 262.)* Sunscreens protect the skin by absorbing and reflecting radiation. Most sunscreens are formulated to protect against UV-B in the range of 290 to 320 nm. The greatest protection is provided by 5% para-aminobenzoic acid (PABA) lotions. Drug-induced photosensitization reactions can be minimized by prescribing sunscreens containing benzophenones. PABA or its derivatives should not be prescribed for persons who have experienced phototoxic reactions with certain drugs, including thiazide diuretics and sulfonamides. In these patients, there may be a cross-reaction with PABA, leading to eczematous dermatitis. Such persons should use benzophenones or opaque sunscreens containing zinc oxide and titanium oxide. Sunscreens containing light-scattering agents such as kaolin may also be used.

480. The answer is D. *(Braunwald, ed 11. pp 684–685.)* The patient presented has a classic case of arthritis secondary to rubella infection. The arthritis is most often seen in young adults although it does occur in children who have been vaccinated with the live, attenuated rubella vaccine. It typically begins soon after the onset of the rash and is self-limiting, usually lasting several weeks. Joint effusions are small and serologic tests are negative. It is a nondestructive arthritis even in patients who have years of recurrent attacks. Other viral infections associated with arthritis include hepatitis B, arboviruses, mumps, infectious mononucleosis, varicella, and adenoviruses.

481. The answer is E. *(Braunwald, ed 11. pp 235–236.)* The course of exfoliative dermatitis is determined by its cause: in patients with generalized skin disease—psoriasis, for example—the disease resolves itself, whereas in systemic disease such as lymphoma, the prognosis is relatively poor. Exfoliative dermatitis may occur as a result of a drug reaction, as a manifestation of a generalized preexisting dermatitis, or in association with systemic disease such as lymphoma and leukemia. Approximately 60 percent of affected patients recover in less than a year, 10 percent have a persistent lesion that does not respond to treatment, and 30 percent die.

482. The answer is E. *(Braunwald, ed 11. p 261.)* Psoralens, used in conjunction with ultraviolet radiation UV-A (320 to 400 nm), are frequently employed in treating psoriasis. Psoralens also have been widely used in treating vitiligo, eczema, and mycosis fungoides. In the presence of psoralen, irradiation with ultraviolet A results

238

in the binding of psoralens to pyrimidine bases in DNA. This reaction leads to inhibition of DNA synthesis followed by cell death. Methoxsalen is given in a dose range of 0.6 to 0.9 mg/kg. Patients who are candidates for this regimen are exposed to a measured dose of ultraviolet radiation following ingestion of the medication. Repeated psoralen–ultraviolet A treatment has been observed to cause disappearance of psoriatic lesions. Possible side effects of this and other types of photochemotherapy include premature aging, cataracts, and skin cancer.

483.   The answer is C. *(Fitzpatrick, ed 3. pp 1328–1334.)* Pyoderma gangrenosum is a progressive ulcerative lesion with a necrotic base and ragged, overhanging borders. It usually begins as a painful, red nodule on the lower extremities. Because the ulceration involves the reticular layer of the dermis and subcutis, scarring occurs on healing. While it is associated with a variety of diseases, it may occur as an illness confined to the skin in 40 to 50 percent of cases. An interesting feature of pyoderma gangrenosum is the susceptibility of the lesion to occur at sites of trauma. The course of pyoderma gangrenosum is highly variable, although when associated with inflammatory bowel disease, it usually parallels the activity of the gastrointestinal dysfunction. Therapy usually involves high doses of corticosteroids.

484.   The answer is D. *(Braunwald, ed 11. pp 415–416.)* The skin findings in the patient presented in the question are classic for scurvy. In the untreated disease, the hair follicles themselves become enlarged and red and, ultimately, hemorrhagic from the proliferation of surrounding blood vessels. None of the other diseases listed in the question produce similar manifestations.

485.   The answer is C. *(Braunwald, ed 11. pp 167, 283, 1437. Fitzpatrick, ed 3. pp 1173–1177.)* Aphthous stomatitis is one of the most common afflictions of the mouth. Between 20 and 50 percent of people suffer occasional or recurrent outbreaks of aphthous ulcers. In one series 50 percent of health professionals questioned stated that they were victims of this disease. Viruses are not cultured from these lesions, although some of them may have a herpetic look to them. The Coxsackie A-16 enterovirus does produce lesions on the lips and oral mucosa that are part of hand-foot-and-mouth disease. A brief prodrome of mild fever, malaise, and gastrointestinal discomfort is followed by the evolution of papulovesicular lesions in the mouth. It appears that aphthous stomatitis is most likely to result from immunological damage to the mucous membranes. Whether this is a true autoimmune phenomenon or a secondary reaction to, for example, streptococcal antigens in the mouth, is not clear. The impression that immune mechanisms may play an important role in this disease is strengthened by the finding that the tendency to develop these ulcers is linked to an HLA A2, B12 haplotype. In addition, a number of immunologic disorders feature aphthous stomatitis. These include Crohn's disease, ulcerative colitis, selective IgA deficiency, pernicious anemia, Behçet's syndrome, and Reiter's syndrome. Although a number of biological response modifiers are being tried, the treatment remains largely symptomatic. Tetracycline suspension held in the mouth for a few minutes before swallowing has been successful for some patients. The lesions may be less painful and heal more rapidly if a steroid in a paste vehicle that will adhere to the oral mucosa is applied to the lesions.

486. The answer is C. *(Braunwald, ed 11. pp 1594–1595.)* Mycosis fungoides, a lymphoma of the skin, can pass through several stages. The first is a diffuse erythroderma and exfoliative dermatitis. In the second phase, plaques develop, and in the third phase, tumors and nodules are found. Not everyone who has exfoliative dermatitis has mycosis fungoides. Exfoliative dermatitis has other causes such as psoriasis, drug reactions, seborrheic dermatitis, and pityriasis rubra pilaris. Erythema multiforme and pemphigus produce blisters. Angiokeratoma corporis diffusum (Fabry's disease) exhibits unusual capillaries in the skin, especially in the groin and eye, and may cause fatal renal disease. Atrophoderma of Pasini and Pierini is an atrophic disease virtually impossible to confuse with an erythroderma.

487. The answer is C. *(Braunwald, ed 11. pp 234–235.)* The patient discussed in the question has an advanced stage of pemphigus vulgaris, a disease that is fatal unless properly treated with prednisone. The drug should be given orally, 100 mg daily or more. When affected patients have improved, the dose can be lowered and methotrexate can be added to minimize the need for oral steroids. However, low-dose steroids or immunosuppressive agents early in the course of pemphigus are often unavailing. Approximately 30 percent of patients having this disease die from complications of treatment; of the survivors, many eventually dispense with medication entirely and lead normal lives.

488. The answer is C. *(Braunwald, ed 11. pp 689–691.)* Most patients who have herpes zoster (shingles) are basically healthy and remain so. However, the disease occurs in 25 percent of patients who have lymphoma, Hodgkin's disease in particular. An affliction chiefly of adulthood, shingles arises from endogenous varicella virus that has lain dormant since the time of its original manifestation as chickenpox. Thus shingles—unlike chickenpox, which is caused by the same virus—is acquired not exogenously but from within. Children who have not been exposed to varicella-herpes zoster virus, when exposed to shingles, can develop chickenpox. There is no documented evidence that shingles is directly transmittable. Unlike herpes simplex, herpes zoster rarely recurs.

489. The answer is E. *(Braunwald, ed 11. pp 1794–1795.)* Lichen simplex is not associated with diabetes mellitus. Disseminated granuloma annulare, however, is frequently the first sign of the disease, and necrobiosis lipoidica diabeticorum and lipoatrophy are virtually pathognomonic signs. Atrophic brown macules, termed diabetic dermopathy, also are classic manifestations of diabetes.

490. The answer is B. *(Fitzpatrick, ed 3. pp 843, 914.)* Becker's nevus is an acquired lesion, occurring most commonly in men, that usually appears in the second or third decade. It most frequently occurs on the shoulder and lower back, is typically light to dark brown in color, and is rarely pruritic. Localized hypertrichosis is common and malignant degeneration does not occur. The other lesions are all present at birth and none are associated with hypertrichosis.

491. The answer is C. *(Braunwald, ed 11. pp 166–167.)* The patient presented in the question probably has aphthous ulcers, lesions that frequently are misdiagnosed as herpes simplex. Herpes tends to cause a group of shallow, round ulcers, frequently beginning as blisters and having a red or yellowish color at the base. These lesions can recur but usually not as often as aphthae. The cause of aphthae is unknown; repeated cultures for viruses, mycoplasmata, and other pathogens have been negative. Moreover, attempts to treat the lesions with antibiotics have been unsuccessful. Topical steroids, while not curative, may be palliative. Topical anesthetics may provide symptomatic relief.

492. The answer is B. *(Braunwald, ed 11. p 283.)* Psoriatic lesions occur quite frequently on the scalp as well as on the elbows, knees, and sacrum. The scalp lesions are sharply demarcated, as are those on the rest of the skin. These sharply demarcated margins differentiate psoriasis from seborrheic dermatitis, which also commonly affects the scalp. Since the scales may be anchored by hair, they may "heap up" so that localized accumulations are usually felt. In contrast, seborrheic dermatitis does not produce this degree of accumulation; instead, it produces a diffuse, scaly erythema. Hair loss does not usually occur in psoriasis unless the hair is removed by excessive scratching of the lesions.

493. The answer is B. *(Fitzpatrick, ed 3. pp 640–641.)* In the patient presented in the question, the most probable cause of hair loss is normal postpartum telogen effluvium. In the first trimester of pregnancy, telogen hairs (resting hairs) constitute a normal 15 to 20 percent of all hair; later in pregnancy, the telogen hair count may drop to 10 percent. This means that many follicles that normally would have reached the end of their active (anagen) phase are still present at parturition. Telogen counts rise quickly in the postpartum period, sometimes reaching 30 to 40 percent of total hair. Telogen lasts approximately 3 months. At the end of this period, there is abnormally heavy shedding while a normal telogen-to-anagen hair ratio is reestablished. A patient who presents with hair loss should be carefully examined for circular bald spots that might indicate alopecia areata or trichotillomania. Trichotillomania, which is loss of hair from pulling, usually causes bald areas with severed hair roots at their bases. Hypothyroidism and hypervitaminosis can both cause alopecia, but there is no reason to suspect them in this patient.

494. The answer is D. *(Braunwald, ed 11. pp 244–245.)* A number of conditions are characterized by a generalized pruritus in the absence of recognizable skin lesions. Hyperthyroidism, carcinoid syndrome, and pruritus of pregnancy often are associated with cholestasis, which may be overt; affected patients may manifest jaundice or merely an elevation of serum alkaline phosphatase and bile acids. Syphilis causes a plethora of skin lesions—notably macules or papules in secondary syphilis. Pruritus in the absence of skin lesions is extremely rare in patients who have syphilis.

495.   The answer is C (2, 4). *(Fitzpatrick, ed 3. pp 1078–1084.)* In the patient presented, the epidemic form of Kaposi's sarcoma is described. Patients typically present with widespread skin lesions and frequently with lymph node and mucosal involvement. In advanced disease, only the brain is spared of lesions. Despite the fact that they are radiosensitive, there is no curative treatment for Kaposi's sarcoma. Chemotherapy has been disappointing, as well, as all patients who respond relapse when therapy is discontinued. All this is in contrast to the Kaposi's sarcoma found in people from tropical Africa and in older persons of Eastern European origin in whom mucosal and lymph node involvement is rare, the response to therapy is excellent, and the clinical course is frequently indolent.

496.   The answer is E (all). *(Braunwald, ed 11. pp 1638–1643. Fitzpatrick, ed 3. pp 1691–1692.)* The porphyrias are a group of diseases that result from abnormalities in heme biosynthesis, both congenital and acquired. Variegate porphyria usually presents in the second or third decade and is characterized by the excretion of large amounts of coproporphyrin and protoporphyrin in the urine. The clinical picture involves acute attacks of abdominal pain and neuropsychiatric dysfunction along with skin lesions. Drugs, such as barbiturates, anticonvulsants, and anesthetics may precipitate attacks of porphyria. Treatment of this disorder involves both glucose and hematin infusions. Porphyria cutanea tarda, on the other hand, is characterized by the increased urinary excretion of uroporphyrin and is commonly associated with alcoholic liver disease and hepatic iron overload; the incidence of diabetes mellitus is increased, as well. The clinical presentation does not include attacks of abdominal pain or neuropsychiatric symptoms; the cutaneous lesions, however, are indistinguishable from those in variegate porphyria. They include vesicles and bullae in areas susceptible to trauma, hyperpigmentation of the face and hands, facial hypertrichosis, and depigmented scars. Treatment of porphyria cutanea tarda involves abstention from alcohol and frequent phlebotomy.

497.   The answer is E (all). *(Braunwald, ed 11. pp 1588–1590.)* When no obvious cause for migratory thrombophlebitis is present, especially when that phlebitis involves areas other than the pelvis, a physician should be suspicious about an underlying malignancy. Often the phlebitis can precede the clinical symptoms and signs of a malignancy by many months. Although carcinoma of the pancreas is the most common tumor with which it is associated, it is by no means the only one. It is unusual to find an operable lesion associated with this sign, so the prognostic significance of the association is grave. Pulmonary embolism is an all-too-common complication.

When epidermal atrophy and hyperkeratosis are associated, the skin appears dry and the stratum corneum sheds rhomboidal scales. In the absence of a family history of this disorder, its development strongly suggests the possibility of an underlying lymphoma. Hodgkin's disease has been the most common malignancy associated with ichthyosis.

The increased hair growth associated with the condition hypertrichosis lanugosa is distinctive. The hair is extremely fine with a silky texture and lightly pigmented. Growth may occur on the trunk, arms, and legs, but the most common sites are the face and ears. Although it can be difficult to differentiate this lanugo proliferation from the effects seen in women with disorders of male sex hormones, the more florid forms of this syndrome are easily recognized. The mechanisms for the production of the hair growth are unclear, but there is a strong association with cancer involving the breast, bladder, lung, gallbladder, colon, and rectum.

Pachydermoperiostosis refers to the condition of hypertrophic osteoarthropathy combined with skeletal changes that are suggestive of acromegaly. The skin of the arms, hands, and legs is markedly thickened as are the facial folds. Just as hypertrophic osteoarthropathy is common in lung cancer, so this extended syndrome is most commonly associated with that disease. Less commonly an acquired form of pachydermoperiostosis is seen with repeated pulmonary infections and hepatic disease. It thus seems to fall into the same group of syndromes in which one may see clubbing of the fingers.

498. The answer is C (2, 4). *(Fitzpatrick, ed 3. pp 654–658.)* Pits are the most common lesion of psoriatic nails and actually represent psoriatic lesions located in the matrix of the nail bed. As the nail plate emerges from the proximal nail fold, the keratotic plug falls off and a pit is formed. The pits typically vary in size, shape, and depth. In alopecia areata, nail pits commonly form in transverse rows.

499. The answer is B (1, 3). *(Braunwald, ed 11. p 1589. Fitzpatrick, ed 3. pp 739–740.)* The patient described has Bowen's disease, or squamous cell carcinoma of the skin in situ. Arsenical exposure has been implicated as causative in most, if not all, cases of the disease. While most lesions do not become invasive and only 2 percent metastasize, their importance lies in their association with gastrointestinal, genitourinary, and pulmonary carcinomas. The risk of an associated neoplasm is particularly high when Bowen's disease occurs on parts of the body not usually exposed to sunlight. The development of a visceral neoplasm may occur many years after the onset of the skin lesion, and examinations for visceral cancer, therefore, should be done at intervals. The lesions should be surgically excised or treated by various methods of local destruction.

500. The answer is A (1, 2, 3). *(Fitzpatrick, ed 3. pp 1874–1882.)* Reiter's syndrome is characterized by arthritis, urethritis, and conjunctivitis occurring predominantly in men between the ages of 15 and 35. Mucocutaneous lesions occur in the majority of patients. Keratoderma blenorrhagica begins as brownish-red macules that develop into hyperkeratotic papules, which may coalesce; these lesions occur mainly on the palms and soles, although any part of the body may be involved. Circinate balanitis occurs on the glans penis as dry, crusting plaques in circumcised men and as shallow, painless ulcers in those uncircumcised. The oral lesions are painless ulcers found on the tongue and hard palate. All lesions heal without scarring.

Bibliography

Adams RA, Victor M: *Principles of Neurology,* 3rd ed. New York, McGraw-Hill, 1985.

Almy TP, Howell DA: Diverticular disease of the colon. *N Engl J Med* 302:324–331, 1980.

Arieff AI, Defronzo RA: *Fluid Electrolyte and Acid-Base Disorders.* New York, Churchill Livingstone, 1985.

Berk JE, et al (eds): *Bockus Gastroenterology,* 4th ed. Philadelphia, WB Saunders, 1985.

Blandy J: *Urology.* St. Louis, CV Mosby, 1976.

Bozymski EM, Herlihy KJ, Orlando RC: Barrett's esophagus. *Ann Intern Med* 97:103–107, 1982.

Braunwald E, Isselbacher KJ, Petersdorf RG, et al (eds): *Harrison's Principles of Internal Medicine,* 11th ed. New York, McGraw-Hill, 1987.

Bukowskyj M, Nakatsu K, Munt PN: Theophylline reassessed. *Ann Intern Med* 101:63–73, 1984.

CA: Guidelines for the cancer-related check-up: Recommendations and rationale. 30:194, 1980.

Case Records of the MGH case 2-1988. *N Engl J Med* 318:100–109, 1988.

Centers for Disease Control, Department of Health and Human Services: Immune globulins for protection against viral hepatitis, recommendations of the immunization practices advisory committee. *Ann Intern Med* 96:193–197, 1982.

Chopra S, Griffin PH: Laboratory tests and diagnostic procedures in evaluation of liver disease. *Am J Med* 79:221–230, 1985.

Chow AW, Jenesson PJ: Pharmacokinetics and safety of antimicrobial agents during pregnancy. *Rev Infect Dis* 7:287–313, 1985.

Eisen HN: *Immunology,* 2nd ed. Hagerstown, Harper & Row, 1980.

Fauci AS, Haynes BF, Katz P, et al: Wegener's granulomatosis: Prospective clinical and therapeutic experience with 85 patients for 21 years. *Ann Intern Med* 98:76–85, 1983.

Felig P, Baxter JD, Broadus AE, Frohman LA: *Endocrinology and Metabolism.* 2nd ed. New York, McGraw-Hill, 1987.

Fishman AP: *Pulmonary Diseases and Disorders,* 2nd ed. New York, McGraw-Hill, 1988.

Force RA, Shizal HM: The assessment of malnutrition. *Surgery* 88:17, 1980.

Fitzpatrick TB, Eisen A, Wolff K, et al: *Dermatology in General Medicine,* 3rd ed. New York, McGraw-Hill, 1987.

Forrester JS, Diamond G, Chatterjee K, et al: Medical therapy of acute myocardial infarction by application of hemodynamic subsets. *N Engl J Med* 295:1356–1360, 1976.

Gottlieb JE, Menashe PI, Cruz E: Gastrointestinal complications in critically ill patients: The intensivist's overview. *Am J Gastroenterol* 81:227–238, 1986.

Greenberger PA, Patterson R: Diagnosis and management of allergic bronchopulmonary aspergillosis. *Ann Allergy* 56:444–448, 1986.

Grieco MH, Meriney DK: *Immunodiagnosis for Clinicians: Interpretation of Immunoassays.* Chicago, Year Book Medical, 1983.

Gross NJ: Pulmonary effects of radiation therapy. *Ann Intern Med* 86:81–92, 1977.

Guenter CA, Welch MH (eds): *Pulmonary Medicine,* 2nd ed. Philadelphia, JB Lippincott, 1982.

Hanifer JM: Basic and clinical aspects of atopic dermatitis. *Ann Allergy* 52:386–393, 1984.

Heffner JE, Miller KS, Sahn SA: Tracheostomy in the ICU, parts I and II. *Chest* 90:269–273, 430–435, 1986.

Hein JJ, et al: The value of the electrocardiogram in the differential diagnosis of a tachycardia with a widened QRS complex. *Am J Med* 64:27–33, 1978.

Hess AD, Esa AH, Colombani PM: Mechanisms of action of cyclosporine: Effect on cells of the immune system and on subcellular events in T cell activation. *Transplant Proc* 20 (no. 2, suppl. 2):29–40, 1988.

Hoeprich PD, et al (eds): *Infectious Diseases: A Modern Treatise of Infectious Processes,* 3rd ed. Philadelphia, Harper & Row, 1983.

Holmes KK, Mardh PA, Sparling PF, Wiesner PJ: *Sexually Transmitted Diseases.* New York, McGraw-Hill, 1983.

Hoshino PK, Gaasch WH: When to intervene in chronic aortic regurgitation. *Arch Intern Med* 146:349–352, 1986.

Hurst JW, Logue RB, Rackley CE, et al (eds): *The Heart,* 6th ed. New York, McGraw-Hill, 1986.

Lance JW: Headache. *Ann Neurol* 10:1–10, 1981.

Lees AJ, Stern GM: Sustained bromocriptine therapy in previously untreated patients with Parkinson's disease. *J Neurol Neurosurg Psychiatry* 44:1020, 1981.

Levy MB, Fink JN: Hypersensitivity pneumonitis. *Ann Allergy* 54:167–171, 1985.

Mandel WJ: *Cardiac Arrhythmias: Their Mechanisms, Diagnosis and Management,* 2nd ed. Philadelphia, JB Lippincott, 1987.

Mandell GL, Douglas RG, Bennett JE: *Principles and Practice of Infectious Diseases,* 2nd ed. New York, John Wiley, 1985.

Maxwell MH, Kleeman CR: *Clinical Disorders of Fluid and Electrolyte Metabolism,* 4th ed. New York, McGraw-Hill, 1987.

McCarty GA: Update on laboratory studies and relationships to rheumatic and allergic diseases. *Ann Allergy* 55:421–433, 1985.

Med Lett Drugs Ther: Gonadorelin-synthetic LH-RH. 25:106, 1983.

Meltzer RS, Cees AV, Fuster V: Intracardiac thrombi and systemic embolization. *Ann Intern Med* 104:689–698, 1986.

Miller RD: *Anesthesia,* 2nd ed. New York, Churchill Livingstone, 1986.

Most H: Treatment of parasitic infections of travelers and immigrants. *N Engl J Med* 310:298–304, 1984.

Murray HW, Rubin BY, Masur H, Roberts RB: Impaired production of lymphokines and immune (gamma) interferon in the acquired immune deficiency syndrome. *N Engl J Med* 310:883–889, 1984.

Patel HP, Anhalt GJ, Diaz LA: Bullous pemphigoid and pemphigus vulgaris. *Ann Allergy* 50:144–149, 1984.

Paul WE (ed): *Fundamental Immunology.* New York, Raven Press, 1984.

Peacock M, Robertson WG: Treatment of urinary tract stone disease. *Drugs* 20:225, 1980.

Pirossky B: Intravenous immune globulin therapy in hypogammaglobulinemia—a review. Intravenous immune globulin and the compromised host. *Am J Med Proc Symposium* 3:53–56, March 1984.

Ponticelli C: Prognosis and treatment of membranous nephropathy. *Kidney Int* 29:927–940, 1986.

Powell LW, Bassett ML, Halliday JW: Hemochromatosis: 1980 update. *Gastroenterology* 78:374–381, 1980.

Rackley CE: *Advances in Critical Care Cardiology.* Philadelphia, FA Davis, 1986.

Rawley JD: Human oncogene locations and chromosome aberrations. *Nature* 301:290–291, 1983.

Rohatgi PK, Goldstein RA: Immunopathogenesis, immunology, and assessment of activity of sarcoidosis. *Ann Allergy* 52:316–325, 1984.

Rose BD: *Pathophysiology of Renal Disease,* 2nd ed. New York, McGraw-Hill, 1987.

Sleisenger MH, Fordtran JS: *Gastrointestinal Disease: Pathophysiology, Diagnosis, Management,* 3rd ed. Philadelphia, WB Saunders, 1983.

Somberg JC, Muira D, Keefe DC: The treatment of ventricular rhythm disturbances. *Am Heart J* 111:1162–1176, 1986.

Spark RF, White RA, Hollowing DB: Impotence is not always psychogenic: New insights into hypothalamic-pituitary-gonadal dysfunction. *JAMA* 243:750, 1980.

Spiro HM: *Clinical Gastroenterology,* 3rd ed. New York, Macmillan, 1983.

Spittell JA Jr (ed): *Clinical Vascular Disease.* Philadelphia, FA Davis, 1983.

Sunderrajan EV, Davenport J: The Guillain-Barré syndrome: Pulmonary-neurologic complications. *Medicine* 64:333–341, 1985.

Thomas GS, Lee PR, Franks P, et al: *Exercise and Health: The Evidence and the Implications.* Cambridge, Oelgeschlanger, Gunn & Hains, 1981.

Waldman RJ, Hall WN, McGee H, et al: Aspirin as a risk factor in Reye's syndrome. *JAMA* 247:308–309, 1982.

Williams WJ, Beutler E, Erslev AJ, et al (eds): *Hematology,* 3rd ed. New York, McGraw-Hill, 1983.

Wilson JD, Foster DW: *William's Textbook of Endocrinology,* 7th ed. Philadelphia, WB Saunders, 1985.